DATE DUE

DEMCO 38-297

GARLAND STUDIES ON

THE ELDERLY IN AMERICA

A collection of monographs and dissertations addressing specific problems facing the elderly in a changing America

EDITED BY
STUART BRUCHEY
Columbia University

A Garland Series

PROSPECTIVE PAYMENTS AND HOSPITAL DISCHARGE PLANNING WITH OLDER ADULTS

Cynthia Stuen, DSW

GARLAND PUBLISHING
New York & London
1991

© 1991 by Cynthia S. Stuen
All Rights Reserved

Library of Congress Cataloging-in-Publication Data

Stuen, Cynthia S.
    Prospective payments and hospital discharge planning with older adults / Cynthia Stuen.
        p. cm. — (Garland studies on the elderly in America; 1)
    Includes bibliographical references.
    ISBN 0-8153-0516-8
    1. Hospitals—New York (N.Y.)—prospective payment. 2. Medicare. 3. Aged—Hospital care—New York (N.Y.) I. Title. II. Series.
    [DNLM: 1. Aged. 2. Nurses—New York City. 3. Patient Discharge-economics—New York City. 5. Social Work-organization & administration—New York City. W 275 AN7 S9p]
    RA982.N49S78 1991
    362.1'9897—dc20
    DNLM/DLC
    for Library of Congress   91-30937
                                                                                                               CIP

Printed on acid-free 250-year-life paper

MANUFACTURED IN THE UNITED STATES OF AMERICA

ACKNOWLEDGEMENTS

This research was conducted with the support of a number of individuals and organizations. To all who contributed their time, expertise and support, I am deeply grateful.

A generous doctoral fellowship was provided to me by the Wahrsager Foundation through the kindness of Karel Wahrsager. This award was given as a memorial to her husband, Sigmund Warhsager, who shared her interest in the increasing problems of an aging population, and to honor two dear friends. Ceevah R. Blatman, whose work in the field of aging brought the concerns of this study topic to her attention, and to Ceevah's late husband, Dr. Saul Blatman, whose true compassion and concern for humanity made him unique in the medical profession. I am very appreciative of the support and extraordinary friendship of Ceevah R. Blatman.

Professor Abraham Monk, Director of the Columbia University Brookdale Institute on Aging and Adult Human Development, served as advisor and provided the encouragement and time to complete this study. Thanks also to all the discharge planners in New York City who gave precious time to participate in this research.

Superlatives do not exist to describe the debt of gratitude I owe to my husband, William A. Weisenbach. He did more than his share of caring for our children, Emily Anne and Matthew Lloyd, while also serving as general editor.

Roots are significant and I thank my parents for giving ones that encouraged self confidence and human service.

CONTENTS

Acknowledgements

1. Context for Study 1

2. The Changing Hospital Environment 7
   Health Policies and Legislation 7
   Organizational Settings of
   Hospitals 16
   Professionalization of Social
   Work and Nursing 23
   Evolution of Medical Social Work 28
   Evolution of Nursing 36
   The Role of Discharge Planners 40

3. Research Design and Methodology 49
   Research Questions 50
   Study Hypotheses 54
   Study Population 56
   Data Collection 57
   Data Analysis 60

4. Profile of Hospital Discharge
   Planners 63
   Hospital Auspice and Size 63
   Profile of Respondents 65
   Employment Information 67

5. DRGs and Discharge Planners
   Activities 71
   Current Discharge Planning Tasks 71
   Time Allocation on Discharge
   Tasks 83
   In/Outpatient Populations 88
   Interdisciplinary Team Meetings 90
   Referral Requirements 91
   Case Management Service Needs 92
   Resource Utilization Groupings 96
   Discharge Planner Opinions 98

Advising about Appeals *106*
　　　Appeals of Discharge Decisions *108*

6. Obstacles to Discharge Planning *111*
　　　Readmission Rates Since PPS *113*
　　　Nurses and Social Workers:
　　　Discharge Planning *116*
　　　Priorities for Professional
　　　Preparation *124*
　　　Personnel Changes Due to PPS *128*

7. Conclusions *131*

Epilogue *141*

Bibliography *147*

Appendix: Hospital Site Visit *175*

Chapter 1

CONTEXT FOR STUDY

This study was designed to determine the effects of the new reimbursement methods on the role of discharge planners in New York City acute care hospitals. It examined the task responsibilities of personnel providing discharge planning services to the elderly. It compared the perceptions of nurses and social workers, the two primary professions involved in discharge planning. The new Prospective Payment System of reimbursement to hospitals is applicable to Medicare-eligible patients only; therefore, it is a fiscal experiment principally affecting older adults (United Hospital Fund, 1986).

Significant demographic changes in the older adult segment of the population have taken and will continue to take place throughout the United States. A dramatic proportional increase in the population 75 years of age and older is projected in the United States. The Bureau of the Census projects that by the year 2000, 6.5% of the total population will be over 75 years of age. Since 1960 the proportion of the population over age 65 nationwide has increased from 9.2% to almost 13% (Soldo and Agree, 1988). New York City is no exception, in 1960 those over age 60 constituted 15% of New York City's population; by 1985 this percentage rose to 18.7%. These trends have contributed to the escalation in health care costs, particularly those associated with Medicare. While the incidence of acute conditions decreases with age, older persons have higher rates of chronic illness, injury, disability and restricted activity than the younger population. As a result, older persons make more use of health services and incur greater health related expense.

In particular, older persons use hospitals at 2.8 times the rate of those under age 65, and their average length of stay in the hospital is longer. In 1980, the population aged 65 and over (11% of population) used 38% of all hospital inpatient days (Schwartz, 1982). The average length of a stay during this same time period increased from 9.8 days for those ages 65-74 to 10.8 days for those ages 75-84 and to 11.7 days for those over 85 years of age (Aging America: Trends and Projections, 1984).

Since the introduction of Medicare and Medicaid (Title XVIII and XIX, respectively, of the Social Security Act), the federal contribution to hospital reimbursement has risen from 12.9% in 1966 to 41.2% in 1981 (Caputi and Heiss, 1984). In 1980, approximately 35% of hospitals' net revenues came from Medicare (AHA, 1981) and 74% of Medicare expenditures were disbursed to hospitals (Gibson and Waldo, 1981). Medicare, the principal source of financing for medical care of the nation's elderly and, as such, the dominant influence on patterns of service began to experience extraordinary change in the 1980's after nearly two decades of almost complete policy stasis.

Prospective versus Retrospective Reimbursement

Perhaps the most significant and certainly the most discussed of these changes was the replacement of retrospective, cost-based reimbursement with a Prospective Payment System (PPS) which establishes fixed prices for each of approximately 470 Diagnosis Related Groups (DRGs). (Special note: because DRGs is the common reference for the Prospective Payment System, both terms will be used in this book interchangeably.) Also significant, especially in terms of attempting to evaluate the impact of the DRGs, was the reconfiguration of utilization controls and quality assurance activities under Professional Review Organizations.

Due to a pre-existing waiver of Medicare payment policies which expired December 31, 1985, New York State implemented the new Medicare Prospective Payment System (PPS) of reimbursement on January 1, 1986. Whereas the rest of the country had been exposed to PPS since 1983, New York had been one of four states with a waiver for adopting the Prospective Reimbursement System. Although there have been many anecdotal reports of adverse consequences for individual patients as a result of the introduction of PPS, systematic data were woefully lacking.

4   Prospective Payments and Discharge Planning

A singular study of twenty-two hospital departments of social work in south-central Illinois was done in 1983 documenting anticipated changes for social work relative to the implementation of PPS(Patchner and Wattenberg, 1985). However, the emphasis of research had not focused on the impact this may have on the social worker's role.

Other than in New York, discharge planning is conducted primarily by nurses (Roberti, 1984). In New York, social workers and nurses are involved in the discharge planning functions, however, there is no standard organizational pattern. Discharge planning may be a part of the social work department or a part of the nursing department.

Another significant development, which undoubtedly had an effect on how hospitals and other health care providers plan and implement post hospital care, was New York State's new method of Medicaid reimbursement to nursing homes. Beginning in January 1986, alongside DRG-PPS Medicare reimbursement method for hospitals, Resource Utilization Groups (RUGs) were implemented. Reimbursement for Medicaid eligible patients in nursing homes is now based on the case-mixed indexes of patients derived from an assessment of the facilities' residents compared to a statewide norm.

Study Purpose

This study determined the effect of the new reimbursement method on the role of discharge planners in New York City's acute care hospitals. From the discharge planner's perspective, it served to allay some fears, and substantiate others, relative to the impact of this new fiscal experiment on the post-hospital planning for older adults. It examined the role of social workers and nurses in discharge planning and made recommendations as to the future role of social workers in discharge planning and their training needs at the professional level.

Research Objectives

The major research objectives of this study were:
1. To identify areas of impact associated with the Prospective Payment System as it affects the role of discharge planners in New York City hospitals, documenting the changes, if any, in role status among discharge planners, codifying differences between nurses and social workers performing parallel discharge planning functions, and identifying potential areas of role confusion.
2. To identify the extent to which discharge planners attribute obstacles or opportunities

associated with successful discharge planning of elderly patients to the new Prospective Payment System.
3. To assess, from the discharge planner's viewpoint, any changes attributable to the Prospective Payment System in the following areas: a) organization of discharge planning activities and staffing; b) specific service needs, particularly case management; c) follow-up and monitoring of community resources arranged on behalf of older persons; and d) the patient's right to appeal discharge decisions.

Chapter 2

THE CHANGING HOSPITAL ENVIRONMENT

The background literature for this study encompasses the following four areas: health policy and legislation, the organizational setting of hospitals for service delivery, development of the professions of nursing and social work, and the evolution of discharge planning.

Health Policies and Legislation in the United States

United States health policy has its roots in the Elizabethan Poor Law of 1601. Since most of the colonial settlers came from England, they provided charity based on the model of the English Poor Laws. Beginning in the seventeenth century, citizens recognized they had a responsibility for those among them who were unable to work as a result of physical illness, lunacy, blindness or other physical impairment. Those deemed worthy or deserving received help; however, each individual or family was carefully evaluated to be certain that an infirmity was not the result of sinful behavior (Demos, 1970). Persons of the middle and upper classes had a responsibility to take care of their own. From the 1800's through the early 1900's, the sick and poor were cared for in public institutions. Hospitals for both the physically and mentally ill were organized by physicians and psychiatrists, but these hospitals were primarily for private patients. Until the Depression of the 1930's, the federal government assumed little responsibility

8   *Prospective Payments and Discharge Planning*

for the health care of its people.

The economic crisis of the Great Depression served as a catalyst for governmental intervention. With the passage of the Social Security Act of 1935, social welfare programs shifted from being the responsibility of localities to a national concern. A health insurance program was recommended by the President's Committee on Economic Security which served as a basis for the Social Security Act. Because he feared jeopardizing benefits to the aged, to the unemployed and to children, President Roosevelt did not recommend passage of the health insurance component.

President Truman advocated a national health insurance plan in 1945, but Congress opposed it. This situation remained unchanged during the Eisenhower years when various health plans were promoted but none ever passed. Building hospitals was more palatable than a national health insurance plan and major hospital construction and renovation occurred with funds from the Hill-Burton Act of 1946. The establishment of the Department of Health, Education and Welfare in 1953 provided the structure for the government to promote health programs. It was clear that the retired older adult population could not finance their medical care on the income they received from Social Security nor could the poor, non-aged afford adequate health care.

The Kerr-Mills Act of 1960 increased

the government's involvement in health care for the poor and aged (Davis and Schoen 1978). This legislation expanded medical care services for welfare clients who were recipients of Old Age Assistance. For those not eligible, Medical Assistance to the Aged took care of physician and hospital services. The Kerr-Mills strategy was means-tested and welfare administered. This legislation reflected the two-tier programs of the colonial period where it had its roots, and reinforced the philosophy that health care is a privilege, not a right.

The Great Society era finally saw the successful passage of two landmark pieces of health legislation in 1965. Amendments to the Social Security Act were Title XVIII (Medicare), to meet the costs of medical services to the aged, and Title XIX (Medicaid), to provide health service coverage for the "medically indigent". The new Medicare and Medicaid legislation prompted concern among lawmakers that services needed to be monitored to insure that quality care continued to be economical. The Medicare legislation stipulated that hospitals and extended care facilities (nursing homes) accepting Medicare had to have Utilization Review Plans (Wilson and Neuhauser, 1976). Utilization review committees were composed of physicians and, often, other health professionals, including social workers and nurses. They were set up to monitor admissions and lengths of stay and guard against inappropriate utilization of beds and facilities. This monitoring resulted in additional legislation in 1972, resulting in Professional Standards Review Organizations (PSROs). This legislation which required the Secretary of Health, Education and Welfare (now Health and Human Services) to designate geographical areas in which panels of physicians were to monitor health services. It has had a profound affect on the consumer health care as well as on all health providers (Miller and Rehr 1983, p.90).

The legislation mandating Professional Standards Review Organizations (PSROs), now called Professional Review Organizations (PROs), is relevant for social workers and is summarized by Miller (1983) as follows: first, Medicare and Medicaid are the most predominant sources of payment for the poor and aged, the two largest constituencies that social workers help; second, the Professional Review Organization legislation establishes parameters for social work functions; third, the built-in cost control factors result in mandates to the social workers that their treatment approaches be consistent with the goal of short term stays in hospitals; fourth, medical recording by social workers must additionally be adequate to meet the purposes of medical care evaluation studies and quality assurance programs as required by PRO Legislation;

fifth, the social worker's recordings provide the basis for medical audits through a peer review process that monitors the quality of the worker's professional practice(*); sixth, by mandating a discharge plan for patients, the legislation highlighted a major function for social workers, who have historically been responsible for discharge planning in hospitals (Miller, 1983).

---

*Coulton (1979) takes issue with this mandate of PRO's and questions whether one can judge the quality of service by looking only at what the worker did or whether it is necessary to look at what happened to the client as a result of the service.

12   Prospective Payments and Discharge Planning

"In reality there is no more important function a hospital social worker can perform, no function that requires greater practice skill than fast assessment of patient need, knowledge of community resources, and formulation of a treatment plan, that will sustain and support the planning" (Miller 1983, p.93). If social workers do not do their discharge planning function expeditiously, there are many other health care providers ready and willing to assume the role, most prominently nurses. The final mandate of PROs, are balancing cost control with quality assurance. Miller also maintains that this should be a major concern for social workers. Quality assurance relies on data collection evaluation of services and outcomes. Can discharge planners facilitate the flow of patients to the community, maintain concern for appropriate bed utilization, provide skillful case management services that are of excellent quality to the client within cost constraints? These are the central concerns among discharge planners today.

While the PRO mandate has enhanced efforts to control the spiraling costs of health care, it has proven inadequate, particularly in light of the demographic trend of increasing numbers of elderly persons. In 1983, Congress passed a law that radically changed Medicare's method of payment for inpatient hospital services. The Social Security Amendments of 1983 (Public Law 98-21) mandated an end to cost-based reimbursement by Medicare and initiated a three-year transition to a prospective payment system (PPS) for inpatient hospital services. The system is based on fixed per-case payment rates for patients in over 470 Diagnosis Related Groups (DRG's). PRO's (Professional Review Organizations) now have monitoring, review and appeal functions for admissions to and discharges from acute care hospitals.

DRG's were developed under the guiding principle that "the primary objective in the construction of DRG's was a definition of case type, each of which could be expected to receive similar outputs or services from a hospital." (NCHS, Pokras,1985, p.1). This was accomplished using clinical judgements and statistical procedures that classify patients by measuring resource utilization. In addition to the medical diagnosis and their clinical management, patient's sex and age were included to arrive at the diagnosis-related groupings. To each of these DRG's is assigned length of stay and approximated use of resources. A fixed per case payment rate is established do that the hospital knows at the moment of admission how much reimbursement it will receive for each patient. If a hospital can treat a patient for less than the payment amount, it may keep the unexpended funds. If the treatment costs more, the hospital must absorb the loss.

Prospective payment constitutes a fundamental restructuring of the financial incentives for hospital care and provides a radical change in the way hospital services will be delivered. The new program was gradually implemented across the country. New York, Massachusetts, New Jersey and Maryland, which already had their own cost-containment measure were exempted through December 1985. On January 1, 1986 the Medicare Prospective Payment System went into effect in these last four states.

Over thirty million older adults and disabled persons, the majority of whom are elderly, depend on Medicare to provide health coverage. A report form the General Accounting Office (Office of Technology Assessment, 1985) on the impact of Medicare's new prospective payment system on post-hospital care of older adults revealed the following findings:

-Patients were being discharged from hospitals after shorter lengths of stay and in poorer states of health than prior to DRG's.

-Beneficiaries were confused and upset about their Medicare benefits.

-It was not clear that post-hospital providers, including nursing homes, home health, and community service agencies, were equipped to deal with sicker patients.

-The demand for post-hospital care was expected to increase under DRG's, yet there was already a shortage of nursing home beds for Medicare patients and limited coverage for services under home and community health programs in many areas.

-Greater demand for the non-hospital services that Medicare covers, such as skilled nursing home care and home health, would mean an increase in costs. This cost-shifting from hospitals to community-based programs would mean more out-of-pocket dollars spent by Medicare beneficiaries (Office of Technology Assessment, 1985).

This climate of cost containment placed a renewed emphasis on discharge planning. For older patients leaving the hospital sooner than before, discharge planning became critical. A patient's level of need may be greater, their families may not be prepared to cope. Finances may be more difficult to manage and the community resources inadequate to meet the demands. Those responsible for discharge planning, more often social workers in New York State, are under increasing pressure to get patients out of the hospital as quickly as possible without having the quality or continuity of care suffer. Such demands may be in conflict with the needs of the patient and his/her family (Shulman and Tuzman, 1980; Abramson, 1981). Whether the discharge planner perceives the hospital discharge function as an opportunity for patient adaptation and growth or one of dysfunction and despair may be indicative of how pressured the role is at this point in time. The impact of the cost containment environment on social workers and nurses responsible for discharge planning in hospitals, on their role, function and educational preparation is of timely importance.

Organizational Setting of Hospitals

Health care organizations are complex social structures, ranging from the large, university-affiliated teaching medical centers to small, community hospitals. Social workers, in particular, employed in health care bureaucracies such as hospitals continue to think of themselves as working in host agencies. Although the majority of social workers identify with organizational structures and institutions, including governmental, voluntary and profit-making, it is fact that they do not control most of the organizations which employ them. This latter point is true for nurses also.

Previously, profession and bureaucracy were thought to be antithetical both at the level of structural principles for organizing work and at the level of motivation and compliance (Davis, 1983). Professional/bureaucratic conflict is a common topic in the theory of organizations literature. One theorist considers the two as opposing institutional forms (Scott, 1966). A professional carries out a complete task on the basis of special knowledge acquired through training; therefore, the professional's allegiance is to the company of professionals. A bureaucrat, on the other hand, carries out a set of tasks which must be coordinated with others. Training is often within the organization and supervision is by a hierarchical superior: therefore, loyalty is to the organization. When a professional works in a bureaucracy, conflict occurs in the resistance to bureaucratic rules, standards, supervision and the demand for unconditional loyalty to the host bureaucracy (Scott, 1966). Physicians, nurses and social workers are among the groups which have been considered professional and thus subject to the types of conflict just outlined (Sorenson and Sorenson 1974, Scott 1969, Wilensky 1964).

Social workers and nurses have a dual responsibility: one responsibility is to the employer, and the other to the client. The employer however, sets down the limits of the service which can be rendered and to some extent determines its kind and quality. The institutional setting of a hospital clearly has an impact on the client/practitioner relationship, affecting practitioner autonomy, client control and most recently, cost implications of remaining in the hospital beyond the allowable time frame.

Another contrast unique to social workers is the client's attitude toward the knowledge of the professional's field. In medicine, for example, clients generally know they need the physician's services and that they lack the knowledge and skill to remedy their problem. This may not always be the case in a client's attitude toward the social worker. The reality of the Prospective Payment System may find a shift occurring whereby social workers' and nurses' knowledge relative to discharge planning might become more highly regarded by both the client and the institution.

Other studies have focused on how organizations can be designed to utilize professional skills. Litwak (1961) offers 'models of bureaucracy which permit conflict'. The notion of autonomous and heteronomous professional organizations, based on Max Weber's concepts of autonomy and heteronomy, provides another classification scheme which contrasts social workers and educators with physicians and lawyers. The former group (social workers and educators) are primarily guided and controlled by administrative rules and by supervisors in the organizational hierarchy. On the other hand, physicians and lawyers are guided and controlled more from within by internalized professional norms, expert knowledge and the professional association (Toren, 1969).

It is argued by some that the central feature of a profession is its autonomy, a factor related to, but not a function of, the knowledge base (Friedson, 1970). Etzioni's classification of full-fledged professional organizations, semi-professional organizations, service organizations and non-professional organizations are attempts to specify structural options for the professional (Etzioni, 1964).

More recent empirical data has shown the joint occurrence of bureaucratization and professionalization. In some cases, they are complementary or have made successful accommodations and in others, role occupants combine professional and bureaucratic roles with ease (Benson, 1973, pp.378-9). Dingwall (1976) shifts the focus to the level of the individual and how the professional fares in various settings; in his term, profession is 'accomplished' in interaction.

A critical feature of health care organizations is the variety of occupations and professions on which they depend in fulfillment of their mission. The history of social work in health care is a legacy of struggle to achieve professional identity, competence, and autonomy in such a complex setting, while developing effective services to patients, families, groups and communities (Germain, 1984). The struggle in some settings has been characterized by the lack of recognition from physicians and by rivalry with other professions, particularly nursing. In other settings, there has been recognition given to social workers and a high value placed on their work with patients and families as well as with members of the interdisciplinary team. Social workers and nurses may also be seen as researchers, teachers of health professionals, including medical students, and community liaisons, providing a bridge from the hospital to the community.

Another organizational feature affecting the nature of professional functions and roles is the need for interprofessional collaboration. Team practice has characterized health care organizations for a long time and gives credence to the philosophy of ministering to the whole person who functions in various social and physical environments. It is assumed in team practice that no single profession alone can meet the biopsychosocial needs generated by illness and disability.

Issues of organizational space and time have an impact on the health care professional's practice, and the availability of space and time may be very limited for discharge planners. These limitations can affect service delivery. The worker's space also includes the neighborhood where resources utilized for referrals are located. The discharge planner in a hospital setting needs to balance the internal organization's needs with the external environment, including the community resource providers and the legislative constraints of benefit entitlements. The fiscal constraints of health care provision directly affect the discharge planner in today's hospital setting.

All professions are experiencing public criticism on matters of effectiveness, ethics, and costs. the decline of public trust in the professions became apparent in the 1960's and has continued ever since (Burnham, 1982). Complaints about professional competence, motivations, and the depersonalization of the relationship between client and professional have mounted; hence an increase in the self-help movement. The elderly, ethnic and racial groups, women and consumer-oriented groups have turned to litigation to redress grievances against a variety of professions through malpractice suits (Yarmolinksy, 1978).

Some discharge planners have expressed concern over ethical dilemmas posed by discharge planning work. The twin issues for social workers and nurses in health care are autonomy and dominance by other professions. Will the Utilization Review Coordinator and administration now pressure physicians to discharge as soon as possible in order to not lose money? There may be movement then from the unprofessionally controlled system of health care to a more collaborative, multiprofessional system in which discharge planners definitely experience gains in control and autonomy.

Discharge planning often provides a classic example of the professional conflict-of-interest dilemmas. In the past, many physicians requested discharge planning services just prior to a patient's leaving the hospital. There is not time in this circumstance for a professionally adequate plan to be developed. This type of referral is prescriptive, thus diminishing the discharge planners opportunity to use professional judgment to properly identify and resolve the problem. The worker often feels conflict when there is inadequate time in which to develop a responsible post-hospital plan of care (Dana, 1983). Discharge planners can use the current legislation to insist on the need for the discharge planning process to begin at the time of admission, or preadmission, and thereby force the physicians to plan ahead.

Consumer concerns raise other dilemmas for workers providing discharge planning services (Black and Canavan, 1985). Patients' rights to participate in their own health care decisions and planning for post-hospital care is still a relatively new concept for some health care professionals. The new reimbursement methodology places stringent time limitations on the hospital stay; the discharge planner must 'get the patient out' often without proper time to plan and without regard for the patient's preference. In addition, the discharge planner may feel powerless to argue for additional time in the hospital in order to provide an adequate post-hospital discharge plan. At the same time there is a movement for hospitals to develop their own home care agencies to insure timely service provision to patients discharged from the hospital. Given the influence of all these various factors on the discharge planning function, this may be the opportune time for discharge planners to advocate for the establishment of improved protocols for referral of patients to needed community-based service providers.

The comparison of nurses and social workers who are discharge planners may enlighten educators as to how each profession is socialized and trained to deal with the above mentioned dilemmas. Do nurses experience less or different types of role stress when told 'to get the patient out' than social workers? Social work departments may be forced to prove themselves as profit-centered departments in this new era of fiscal constraints. Will this force them to abandon the most needy clientele for those who have resources to pay for social services or will it mean that only patients covered by the Prospective Payment System (principally the elderly at this point in time) will be given priority attention?

It has long been known that limited participation in decision-making, ambiguity about job security, poor use of skills and abilities are correlated with job related stresses and job dissatisfaction (Argyris, 1964; Likert, 1961). Attitudes of discharge planners about the new Prospective Payment System are probed and documented in this study.

Professionalization of Social Work and Nursing

Historically the professions referred only to divinity, law, and medicine. "These were generally studied in the Christian universities of Europe beginning in the Middle Ages. In fact, the universities were schools where young men learned to profess Christian learning and to apply it to the three 'learned' fields" (Hughes et al, 1973, p.1).

Carr-Saunders has categorized and ranked professions by the type and amount of knowledge upon which they are based. Medicine and law (along with the ministry) are classified as "the established professions" whose practice is based upon protracted learning of theoretic knowledge. Social work, nursing, librarianship and education are classed as "semi-professions," where study of a theoretic nature is replaced with the acquisition of technical skill (Carr-Saunder, 1955).

It has been seventy years since Abraham Flexner (1915) asked the question, "Is Social Work a Profession?" Briefly stated, Flexner's criteria at that point in time for professional status were: 1) Activities are intellectual in character, 2) derived from science, 3) ideas of learning worked into practice, 4) definitive in purpose, 5) brotherhood (sic) in nature, 6) tending to be altruistic in motivation (Flexner 1915, p.8). Flexner maintained social work was not a profession because it usually invoked another specialized agency to bring this or that profession into action e.g. medicine or law. He maintained that professions have definite and specific ends but that social work did not; rather, it drew on certain aspects of law, education and other professions. According to Flexner, social work was most concerned with supplementing other professions that fell short of what they should be doing. One could venture to guess, that Flexner would place nursing in the same category.

"Deprofessionalization of Social Work" was the title of a 1972 article by Harry Specht. Specht, agreeing with Herman Stein (1969), charged that social workers have come to recognize that they lack the power to make social changes which they desire but have not scaled down their aspirations or commitment to social change. Specht said that when social workers behaved as advocates, they were little more than clubhouse lawyers or politicians. He declared that one must choose between a commitment to social justice and professional practice (Specht, 1972, p.5).

The rejection of the social action thrust was connected to efforts to upgrade the status of social work. The role of the social worker was to be seen as based upon 'scientific knowledge' and methods acquired by distinctive training, thus protecting it from encroachment by others without proper training (Gurin and Williams, 1973; Toren, 1969).

The 'true professional', according to Moore, deals with specific clients and their welfare is affected by competence and quality of service performed. Professionalism should be regarded as a scale or continuum rather than a cluster of attributes (Moore, 1970). The scale includes, 1) practice of a full-time occupation as a principal source of income, 2) possession of useful knowledge and skills based on specialized training or education, 3) identification with peers, 4) commitment to a calling, 5) a service orientation, and 6) autonomy (Moore 1970, p.5). These characteristics are not meant to be of equal value but are clusters on a scale. In varying degrees of consensus, social workers and nurses most likely can identify with such criteria.

Goode (1957) puts forth six factors which together make the "community of professions." These are 1) common and lasting sense of identity with the profession, 2) a central core of shared values, 3) an agreed upon set of role definitions, 4) a common language, 5) communal power over individual members, and 6) careful selection of and socialization of new members. Regarding medicine, in the United States from the Colonial Period to 1900 there was very little organized health care; hence, health professionals were not a major issue. Almshouses incarcerated the poor and substituted as hospitals. The first almshouse was established by William Penn in Philadelphia in 1713. Bellevue Hospital in New York City became the second multipurpose - almshouse and included medical care as one of its functions. As early as 1860, it was recognized that someone needed to check patients' homes for conditions which exacerbate illness. The New York Infirmary for Women and Children called this job "sanitary visitor" and it led to a full time "home visitor" position by 1890 (Wallace et al. 1984). Hence it was observed how the charity movement affected not only the dispensing of relief-'not alms but a friend'-but also the delivery of health care.

Dr. Charles P. Emerson of Johns Hopkins was resident physician of the Baltimore Charities Organization Society. He became impressed with the concept of friendly visiting at patients' homes and applied it to the training of medical students. It was the first attempt at training doctors in social service (Wallace et al. 1984, p.5).

Dr. Richard Cabot, Director of the Outpatient Clinic at Massachusetts General Hospital, visited John Hopkins and was very impressed with the physicians as friendly visitors concept. Combined with his previous experience as Director of Boston's Childrens Aid Society, where he came to value the social histories taken by caseworkers, Dr. Cabot hired a social worker for the outpatient department in 1905. He is credited with establishing the first hospital funded social service department in 1919.

Initially social workers in hospitals were faced with hostility from nurses who would restrict their presence in the wards. This tension eased by employing nurses who were experienced in charities organization work as social workers. These nurses did not identify as nurses but rather as caseworkers. Ida Cannon, a nurse hired by Cabot at Massachusetts General Hospital, became very prominent in the newly created field of medical social work. It is noted in the literature that hospital-based nurses were the handmaidens to physicians and felt the role to be far less prestigious than that of social workers who could make social diagnoses (Wallace et al, 1984).

To upgrade one's status from a physician's handmaiden to the more independent professional they perceived social workers to be may be reflected by their eagerness to take on the discharge planning role when some social workers thought it beneath their worth to arrange the concrete services often associated with discharge planning. It is an interesting contrast that social workers have sought to regain the discharge planning role in recent years prompted, perhaps, by awareness that nurses, not paraprofessionals, were eager to assume the discharge planning functions (American Association of Continuity of Care, 1984). The evolution of medical social work and nursing enhances one's understanding of the above phenomenon as presented next.

Evolution of Medical Social Work

Just as relief workers discarded the volunteer approach as unprofessional, medical social workers insisted on paid employment, educational requirements and professional recognition. In 1912, Ida Cannon arranged with Jeffrey Brackett at the Boston School of Social Work (Harvard-Simmons, then Simmons) to begin a one year training program for medical social workers. The training included ten months of practical supervision at Massachusetts General Hospital. In addition, the scheduled lectures and conferences covered the following topics: psychology, mental hygiene, sociology, dietetics, biology, basic medicine, and review of community resources. The New York and Philadelphia Schools of Social Work followed suit and by 1920 had identified minimum educational requirements for medical social work.

In the case of medical social work, the impetus for specialized social work training came from the field of practice not the schools (Gurin and Williams, 1973). In 1932 the American Association of School of Social Work adopted a specific curriculum for medical social work which followed two decades of great debate on generic versus specific training for social workers. However in 1939 the generalists prevailed when social work training expanded to two years and specialized training was lost.

Medical social workers were the first group of social workers to organize professionally. The American Association of Hospital Social Workers was established in 1918. The job of medical social work was given increasing visibility after World War I when great numbers were recruited to work with veterans and their families. The Influenza Epidemic of 1918, and the spread of tuberculosis and venereal disease created a great demand for social workers. Given the difficulty of the job, it was seen as one of responsibility, not choice; it was work that had to be done (Wallace et al. 1984, p.9).

Discharge planning has an uneven history in social work practice. When medical social work began at Dr. Cabot's instigation in 1905, its principal function was to help in post-hospital planning so patients could sustain their health gains.

Social workers who focused on the 'mind' of the patient as the primary mode of intervention began to separate themselves from the medical social workers in 1926. Psychiatric social workers had contempt for medical social workers who concerned themselves only with the social dimensions of patient care. Medical social workers rebutted that they too had expertise in the emotional dimension of patients in order to share in the newly claimed prestige of the psychiatric social workers. From 1920 to 1950, little emphasis was given to the realm of medical-social diagnoses in comparison to the psychological. Sigmund Freud's emphasis on the intrapsychic had a powerful impact on social work and took dominance over the social environment emphasis as described in <u>Community Psychiatry</u> (Meyer, 1948). In many health care settings discharge planning came to be relegated to social workers with less than graduate education on the assumption that it required less knowledge and skill than the counseling function (Germain, 1984).

The American Association of Hospital Social Workers along with other specialized groups of social workers, was absorbed into the National Association of Social Workers in 1955. The Society for Hospital Social Work Directors of the American Hospital Association was formed in 1965. This coincides with the tremendous growth in social work departments necessitated by Medicare and Medicaid legislation passed that same year. The Medicare and Medicaid legislation established a cost-based mechanism of reimbursement for all care required by patients. Hence, hospitals could employ social workers as needed and receive an adequate reimbursement from these funding sources to cover their costs.

A listing of the components of the clinical role in hospital social work follows, discharge planning is listed as one of nineteen components:

> Case finding or social risk screening
> Preadmission planning
> Psychosocial evaluation
> Psychosocial intervention
> Financial assistance
> Case consultation to hospital staff
> Facilitating use of hospital services
> Health education
> *Discharge planning
> Information and referral
> Facilitation of community agency referrals

32   *Prospective Payments and Discharge Planning*

>Case consultation to community agencies
>Utilization Review
>Research
>Program consultation to hospital staff
>Hospital planning
>Program consultation to community agencies
>Community service
>Community health planning

There is a growing recognition of the importance of maintaining and even extending social workers traditional involvement in discharge planning (Shulman and Tuzman, 1980). Many practical suggestions on how social workers can contribute to the hospitals' efforts to prevent patients from staying in the hospital too long without forfeiting their needs and rights are being implemented. One suggestion has focused on early referrals (Boone et al. 1971; Schrager et al. 1978). Others advocate early identification of patients requiring discharge planning and suggest screening patients prior to or during admission procedures (Lurie et al. 1981; Phillips, 1972; Abramson, 1981). To facilitate early involvement there has been some movement toward specialized discharge planning units, discharge planning wards, and specialized skill training for social workers (Krell, 1977; Foster and Brown, 1978; Grossman et al. 1979).

Various medical factors which delay discharge have also been identified. These include chronic illnesses, need for nursing home care, illnesses with unanticipated consequences, and political-economic conditions such as availability of resources (Schrager, 1978; Berkman et al. 1980; Coulton et al. 1982). It is the author's premise that this task has gained increased attention and may consume the majority of a social worker's time in working with older adults.

Discharge planning occupies a great deal of a social worker's time in acute care hospitals (Lurie et al. 1981). The American Hospital Association through its Office on Aging and Long Term Care surveyed its membership and identified hospitals which offer services specifically for older adults. A study of those hospitals (N=689) with specialized services for the elderly reported discharge planning the most frequently offered service (75%). There were a total of twenty-nine services reported by the hospitals. After discharge planning, information and referral was the next highest reported service at 47.6% (Evashwick et al. 1985).

The social work profession today appears to be reemphasizing discharge planning, which is reflected in changing staffing patterns and program development (Lurie et al. 1981). Discharge planning has become an increasingly important component of hospital management and operation over the past decade (Blazyk and Canavan, 1985). It would appear that the social work profession is returning to the model of practice in hospitals first established by Ida Cannon; reuniting the delivery of concrete services and clinical help (Regensberg, 1978).

"Although planning the discharge of a hospitalized patient is often a complicated task that requires interprofessional collaboration, the task has come to have particularly negative meaning for some social workers. There are professional social workers who consider that all of the work connected with discharge planning can be carried effectively by well-trained paraprofessionals. There are other social workers who recognize, value, and use their special clinical competence to handle problems of discharge which require their expertness in helping to resolve conflicts between family members and health care personnel and to reduce other emotional burdens that may arise in planning discharge." (Regensberg, 1978, p.108).

Discharge planning has been viewed by some social workers as a routinized service requiring little skill or expertise (Ullman and Kassebaum, 1961). The curricula of two schools of social work in New York City were examined by Lurie in 1980 as to their course offerings and content related to discharge planning. There was no formal organization of a curriculum that was specifically focused on discharge planning. Five areas of curriculum content that need to be presented to social workers assuming responsibilities in discharge planning were identified by this study, they are: assessment, collaborative assessment, collaborative practice, legislative and regulatory systems, community resources and intervention skills (Lurie et al. 1981).

Lurie and colleagues also surveyed supervisor and student participants in discharge planning programs and found need, in both schools of social work and continuing education programs, for a more focused introduction of discharge planning and the skills required. In addition, the findings suggested that schools of social work need to maintain flexibility in their course content to meet shifts in the practice of discharge planning and that agencies should provide feedback to schools to determine if students are meeting criteria for their first professional experience in discharge planning. The above study is limited by the small sample of supervisors and students affiliated with a modest consortia of agencies. This research study asks both nurses and social workers to assess priorities for graduate curricula in this area.

One final area deserves mention in the evolution of hospital-based social work. The hiring of social workers by non- social workers in hospitals led to a joint committee of the American Hospital Association and National Association of Social Workers in 1976 developing eleven standards for hospital social service. Ten of these standards were accepted by the Joint Commission on Accreditation of

Hospitals in 1979. The one standard not accepted was that an MSW or BSW with MSW supervision/consultant was necessary to head a department of social services in every hospital. The Joint Commission claimed it was a 'restraint of trade' issue...and so the lack of professional recognition continues. In spite of this action by the Joint Commission, most hospital departments of social work, particularly in New York City, do appoint directors prepared at the baccalaureate or masters level.

Evolution of Nursing

Florence Nightengale balanced the elements of good medicine, namely, to fight disease through the application of physical and biological sciences, and the application of behavioral and social sciences to cheer patients. Formal training for nurses was advocated by Florence Nightengale and she founded the Nightengale School in 1860 in London, England. This new school was affiliated with St. Thomas Hospital. The first nursing school in the United States opened in 1873 and was modeled on the Nightengale School.

A note of interest posited by Florence Nightengale with respect to nursing as a 'woman's profession' revealed in the following quote, "...especially hospital nursing, a woman is really in charge of men." (Seymour, 1954, p.321). Ms. Nightengale may not have been pleased with the early evolution of nursing which has often been perceived as the 'handmaidens of physicians'. Ms. Nightengale opposed the registration of nurses in the late 1880's because she felt, "Every woman...has, at one time or another of her life, charge of the personal health of somebody, whether child or invalid- in other words, every woman is a nurse." (Seymour, 1954, p.123).

The education of nurses was almost exclusively hospital based until the late 1940's. Hospitals were the primary employers of nurses therefore it was in their best interest to assume responsibility for preparing them. Nursing educators questioned the hospital's role as an educational institution and leveled the criticism that hospital needs rather than needs of students were a priority in the preparation of nurses (Curran and Metcalf, 1983).

Confusion in role expectations and its attendant type of basic educational preparation dates back to 1948 (Rothweiler, 1986). At that time, two separate groups, the President's Commission on Higher Education and the Committee on the Function of Nursing, issued statements on nursing education. The President's Commission on Higher Education wrote that a semiprofessional nurse's education must aim at developing a combination of social understanding and technical competence. This preparation for second level nursing should include a fair amount of general education for personal development and a technical education that is intensive, accurate and comprehensive enough to give the student a command of marketable abilities (American Nurses Association, 1979).

The Committee on the Function of Nursing, during the same year, stated that the professional nurse should head the nursing team, provide professional counsel and retain supervisory responsibility. However, the Committee failed to make clear whether a diploma or a baccalaureate degree constituted an "adequate education" for professional nurse status as opposed to technical nurse status (Committee on the Function of Nursing, 1948). The license for practical nurses was developed at about the same time. It is understandable that there was role confusion in the nursing profession during its formative period.

In 1960, the American Nurses' Association on recognition of this confusion approved the following goal, "Within the next 20-30 years, the education of professional nursing will be secured in a program that provides intellectual, technical and cultural components of both a professional and liberal education. To this end, the baccalaureate program will be the basic educational foundation for professional nursing (American Nurses' Association, 1979).

The Surgeon General's Consultant Group on Nursing, in 1963, pointed out that there was no consistent differentiation as to levels of responsibility assigned to baccalaureate, technical and practical nurses (DHEW, 1963). The American Nurses' Association responded that a) education for nurses should take place in institutions of higher education; b) minimum preparation for beginning professional practice is a baccalaureate; c) minimum preparation for beginning technical nursing practice should be the associate degree; and d) education for assistants in health care should be short, intensive pre-service programs in vocational education institutions rather than on-the-job (American Nurses' Association, 1964, p.49). As nurses began to delineate their roles based on educational requirements, they drew on social work and other professions for collaboration and guidance (Lysault, 1977; Burling et al. 1956; Schoenberg et al. 1968; Wlaters, 1965).

The discipline of nursing has undergone an identity crisis in the 1960's and 1970's. Depending on the period, nursing has been described as an art, a science, and a profession (Barrow, 1978). The nurse's role has evolved from one of care for the ill in a support role to the physician and has struggled to move to a more independent role. For example, Orem (1980) delineates a diagnostic and prescriptive role for nurses. "The first step of the nursing process is diagnosis and prescription. Diagnosis is an investigative operation that enables nurses to make judgements about existing health care situations and decisions about what can and should be done." (Orem, 1980, p.191). Numerous articles have been written about nurses' interest and quest for autonomy, that freedom to make discretionary and binding decisions consistent with one's scope of practice and freedom to act on decisions (Batey and Lewis, 1982). This movement toward more autonomous practice bears out Ida M. Cannon's theory that nurses envied the independence of social workers in their ability to make social diagnoses (Cannon, 1913).

The Role of Discharge Planners

Discharge planning has achieved greater importance in the hospital with the current changes in the fiscal and regulatory climate (Schreiber, 1981). Social workers are moving ahead to redefine and regain the discharge planning function that many of them relinquished, primarily to nurses in the past (Germain, 1984). Bailis (1985) suggests social workers have not been aware that discharge planning offers a potential raison d'etre to social work departments that psychotherapy alone does not. Social workers may feel a role conflict between their colleagues in social work who denigrate discharge planning and the hospital physicians and administrators who value their role. The prospective payment mechanism, according to some leaders in this field, provides an opportunity for social workers to upgrade their status as timely discharge of patients is of the utmost importance to the hospital for its fiscal survival (Coulton, 1982; Kane, 1983).

Rademaker (1982) states that nursing's broad functional base is being eroded by encroachment from other occupational groups. Specifically the areas of discharge planning and counseling are mentioned as being encroached on by social workers. A valued position in the multidisciplinary health care setting is sought by nursing and a strategy of 'demonstrating competence' is suggested as the means to obtain it. "A valued position is extremely important as new occupations define their turf, in part, by attempting to encroach on nursing's turf" (Singleton and Nai 1984, p.20).

Stepping outside the hospital for a moment, historically, the community health nurse was the dominant and often only provider of home health care. Social workers are a relatively new addition to home health agencies and have contributed to turf conflict in this arena (Lowe, 1978). It is suggested that as the population ages and the cost of institutionalization increases, more and more people will need services in their home and that a variety of professionals will be necessary (Fessler and Adams, 1985).

Recognition of turf issues between social workers and nurses in hospitals is also well documented in the literature as reflected by titles such as: "Case Material: A Meeting Ground for Nurses and Social Workers" (Lipeles, 1959); and "Burying the Turf Issue" (Isenberg and Cramand, 1986).

A study conducted by S.S. Robinson in the 1960's addressed the issue of, "Is There a Difference?" in the perception of public health nurses and social workers in each others specific and overlapping functions. Robinson's study determined the extent of agreement among public health nurses and social workers about their professional activities. She measured which functions they considered to be appropriate to their profession only; which they would assign to the other profession; which they consider require the contribution of both for the most satisfying outcome; and which they think could be performed by either public health nurses or social workers. The findings revealed the greatest agreement was in the number of activities requiring a collaborative effort, although the majority in each group would collaborate on relatively few activities. One striking finding of this study was that the more education either professional had, the less likely they were to indicate collaborative activities (Robinson, 1967). The research framework from the Robinson study has been adapted in the present research study providing a comparison of nurses and social workers in the acute hospital setting conducting discharge planning activities.

More attention is being given to the professional demands of discharge planning. A number of articles in professional social work and nursing journals have been published which emphasize the importance of discharge planning (Kane, 1980; Schreiber, 1981; Coulton et al. 1982; and Kulys, 1983; Piper, 1983; Houston and Cadenhead, 1986; Toth, 1984; Schaeffer, 1984a, 1984b, 1984c; and Rasmusen, 1984).

In an editorial in Health and Social Work, Kane wrote that if social workers can demonstrate an ability to facilitate timely discharges, their place in the hospital may be strengthened by the introduction of DRGs. She also stressed the importance of early case finding and high risk screening for discharge planning efficiency (Kane, 1983). It will be of interest to document if discharge planners are able to do their own case-finding and whether they begin the discharge planning process prior to admission for patients admitted for non-emergent treatment. Nursing also stresses the importance of early screening in the discharge planning process and there is a proliferation of literature documenting the importance of 'screening tools' (Knight, 1986; Alami and Urtel, 1986; and Rasmusen, 1986).

Several obstacles to good discharge planning are cited in the literature. Foremost is the lack of adequate resources to meet the needs of patients ready for discharge from acute care hospitals. Often planning is based on availability of governmental programs and financial resources. For patients unable to return to their own home, the problem of identifying and finding space in an appropriate alternative facility is sometimes a major obstacle (Lurie and Rosenberg, 1984).

If patients and their families are suffering/coping with an acute medical episode which requires hospitalization, often there is inadequate time to deal with the issues of illness and the reality of post-hospital care. A situation such as this exacerbates the conflict felt by discharge planners who are caught between the demands of the hospital(employer) pressuring for speedy discharge planning, and the need of patient and/or family for more time for the planning process.

An obstacle commonly attributable to interdisciplinary practice is role blurring which may occur when 'everyone' is focused on 'getting the patient discharged.' Extreme role specialization can also occur which could leave the discharge planner without general or overall biomedical data needed to effectively plan for post hospital care.

Social workers and nurses are also under pressure to address the need for their professions to contribute to the profitability and fiscal stability of the hospitals they serve (Schreiber, 1981; Marshall, 1984; Vollard, 1983; Grimaldi, 1983; and Hamilton, 1984).

The discharge planning function is defined by the Committee on Discharge Planning of the Society for Hospital Social Work Directors of the American Hospital Association as follows:

"Successful discharge planning is a centralized, coordinated, interdisciplinary process that ensures a plan for continuing care for each patient. It reflects both the patient's sand family's internal and external social, emotional, medical and psychological needs and assets. It recognizes that the transition from the hospital is often more threatening than the actual hospitalization and a plan must be developed to both provide for a continuum of care and address the patient's immediate needs following discharge. It is the clinical process by which health care professionals, patients, and families collaborate to ensure that patients have access to services that enable to regain, maintain, and even improve the level of functioning achieved in the hospital" (Cochrane et al. 1980, p.3). The committee later added:

How patients are discharged from the hospital and the kinds of after-care they receive is the concern of many health care professionals. But, the skills required to help patients and families identify their goals and fully use their own strengths, as well as translate these into realistic, coordinated plans, are basic social work skills...The discharge planner must provide emotional support to the patient and family, both before and during the transition from the hospital; must assist the family in exploring options for adjusting their finances; must help the patient adjust to a new self-image; must coordinate the community resources that support the transfer from the hospital and that provide post-hospital care; and must refer the family to support and education groups which will continue to assist them (Cochrane 1981).

The emergence of discharge planning as a separate 'profession' can be documented by two separate movements. One is the founding of a new national organization for discharge planning professionals and the other is passage of state regulations governing this discipline.

In 1975, the discharge planning association in Brooklyn, New York wrote a position paper on discharge planning which received national attention when it was featured in both <u>RN Magazine</u> and <u>The American Journal of Nursing</u>. By 1980, the Brooklyn group of discharge planners expanded to become the Association of Discharge Planning Coordinators in New York City. The Brooklyn group conducted two national surveys which revealed that professionals involved in discharge planning felt no other organization was meeting their needs and supported the concept of a new national organization. Planning sessions with both the American Hospital Association and the National Association of Quality Assurance Providers resulted in the birth of the American Association of Continuity of Care (AACC) in September, 1982. The structure of AACC embraces the concept of networking to help educate and support discharge planners who work as part of a multidisciplinary team. That continuity of care is an essential component of the health care delivery system; that every patient has a right to quality, coordinated discharge planning, and that discharge planning is a holistic health approach that is centered on the patient and family are the basic premises of the AACC organization (Craig, 1985).

The second movement involves 1986 revisions to the Public Health Law, Subchapter A (Medical Facilities-Minimum Standards) of Chapter V, Title 10 (Health) of the official Compilation of Codes, Rules and Regulations of the State of New York. Specifically, each hospital shall have in operation an organized discharge planning program...to meet the patient's post-discharge needs. It further requires that there shall be a discharge planning coordinator who has been delegated the responsibility for the execution of the organized discharge planning program. the discharge planning coordinator is defined as someone who shall be a "qualified social worker, a community health nurse with at least one year of experience working with non-institutional health care services or human services agencies." A qualified social worker is someone who has graduated from an accredited social work professional school.

This chapter has documented the health legislation and policies which gave birth to a Prospective Payment System that places a very high premium on 'expeditious discharges' from acute care hospitals. Social workers and nurses in their struggles to gain professional recognition and autonomy have begun to seize the discharge planning function in a new way, heretofore not documented in the literature of either profession. This study attempted to document the discharge planning activities as conducted in New York City hospitals and better understand the early impact which the Prospective Payment System was having on the role of the discharge planner. it identifies the role changes attributable to the Prospective Payment System and how nurses and social workers may vary in their approach to the critical area of discharge planning functions with older adults.

Chapter 3

RESEARCH DESIGN AND METHODOLOGY

Prior to the development of the research protocol, a series of exploratory and fact-finding consultations were conducted with various individuals involved in discharge planning work. Among them were discharge planning coordinators, utilization review coordinators, directors of hospital social work, supervisory level and line workers in social work, supervisory level and line workers in social work departments responsible for discharge planning, and discharge planning unit/department personnel. Two organizations, were involved at the very early stage of research question identification and remained involved throughout the study implementation. The two organizations were the association of Discharge Planners in New York City and the New York Society for Hospital Social Work Directors. The executive committees of both groups were given presentations on the study in Fall, 1985 and gave support to its implementation in 1986.

The primary data source of this study of discharge planners in New York City acute care hospitals was derived from a mail survey based on a questionnaire specifically designed for this study. A second data source was a site visit to an acute care hospital to provide a dynamic documentation of the discharge planning process. The site visit was conducted by the researcher with interviews involving the following departments or units: social work, discharge planning, utilization review, quality assurance, geriatric primary care clinic, and administration. Questions probed at the case study hospital were guided by the survey data analysis. Data from the site visit are reported in the appendix.

Research Questions

Based on a review of the discharge planning literature and consultation with representatives in hospitals familiar with discharge planning, the following eleven questions served as a guide for the development of a survey instrument.
Question I. *What are the current task responsibilities of discharge planners in acute care hospitals?*

Nineteen activities were culled from the social work and nursing literature and current providers of discharge planning services which reflect a composite for discharge planners. Each activity was rated on a five point Likert scale as to the frequency of performance.

Additional questions gathered information on the size of the caseload for discharge planners, the percentage of elderly among that caseload and information on high risk screening and follow-up activities.

Question II. *Has the implementation of the Prospective Payment System changed any of the discharge planning duties and responsibilities?*

The nineteen discharge planning activities previously identified were repeated and the respondent asked to indicate how the time spend on each function had been affected as a result of the new Prospective Payment legislation. A five-point Likert scale was utilized for responses.

If the answer was yes, a further contingency question was asked to determine if this was a change since DRGs went into effect.

Question III. *How have discharge planners' reacted to the new Prospective Payment System?*

A thirteen item scale was constructed based on a model developed by Patchner and Wattenberg (1985). They developed it for use in a survey study with Directors of Social Work in Central Illinois hospitals to assess anticipated changes and opinions relative to forthcoming implementation of the Prospective Payment System. The areas covered were role status, service organization, coordination and delivery. The items were rated on a five-point Likert type scale.

Question IV. *Has the discharge planner's responsibility for advising patients about their right to appeal discharge decisions been affected by the Prospective Payment System?*

Five questionnaire items addressed this concern; two related directly to the appeals mechanism and three questions were more general, concerning DRG-information requested by patients.

Question V. *What is the Discharge planner's perception of the reasons for patient appeals to discharge decisions?*
Three questions assessed this concern and had fixed-frequency response choices.

Question VI. *In what ways do discharge plans sometimes go awry under the new DRG system?*
This was an open-ended question allowing respondents to write their opinions without confinement. The responses were later categorized into nine groups.

Question VII. *How frequently do patients and their kin/kith present obstacles to the discharge planning process?*
Six obstacles attributable to a patient's ability to cooperate with discharge planning were identified, in addition to six obstacles attributable to a patient's support network and its ability to cooperate with discharge planning.

Question VIII. *Have discharge planners noticed a higher rate of readmission of elderly patients since the Prospective Payment System went into effect and to what do they attribute the readmission?*
A single contingency question ascertained if discharge planners felt there was a higher rate of readmission. If discharge planners replied affirmatively, a rank ordering of the

most frequently observed factors (a fixed-choice response) to readmission was obtained.

Question IX. *How do social workers and nurses perceived the appropriate discipline for performing parallel discharge planning functions?*

An adaptation of the research design used in a study of public health nurses and social workers conducted by S. S. Robinson (1967) was applied to discharge planners, some of whom are nurses, and others social workers. Respondents were asked to indicate whether one discipline, *nursing* or *social work,* is best suited to perform the function, whether *either* discipline might effectively perform the function, or whether a *collaborative* effort (one in which both nurses and social workers are needed for optimum results) is best. Throughout the data analysis, there are comparisons of nurses and social workers in their responses to questions and when significant variance occurs, it has been reported.

Question X. *What recommendations would discharge planners make for shaping their professional discipline curriculum, to meet the needs of discharge planners?*

Respondents were first asked if they had a professional discipline. If the reply was affirmative, respondents were asked how adequately their professional school had prepared them for discharge planning responsibilities. Respondents were then asked to place themselves in the position of advising their professional school regarding curriculum priorities.

Eight types of skills which discharge planners need were culled from the literature and meetings with key informants. Respondents were asked to rank each skill area on a five-point scale.

Question XI. *Have there been any personnel changes in the hospitals' discharge planning staff attributable to the Prospective Payment System?*

This question ascertained whether there had been any change and the nature of the change.

Study Hypotheses

Several of the critical questions lend themselves to hypotheses.
1. Ho: The Prospective Payment System has not changed the discharge planning tasks among acute care hospital discharge planners.
2. Ho: Social Workers and nurses do not differ in how they identify time-allocation changes due to the Prospective Payment System.
3. Ho: Discharge planners perceive no change in their value the hospital as a result of DRGs.
4. Ho: Social workers and nurses do not differ in perception of DRG-induced role changes, if any.
5. Ho: Discharge planners do not view their role as being responsible for

advising patients of appeal information.
6. Ho: Discharge planners are not aware of reasons or outcomes of appeals decisions.
7. Ho: There is no agreement concerning collaboration between social workers and nurses for achieving optimal discharge planning.

Survey Instrument

The survey questionnaire was constructed with both closed and open-ended items as reflected by the elaboration of each of the eleven critical questions. The survey sought to elicit factual and attitudinal data from discharge planners who work with older adults in acute care hospitals in New York City.

A pretest of the survey instrument was conducted at four acute care hospitals outside New York City; three in Westchester County and one in Nassau County. The pretest was conducted with social workers and nurses representative of supervisory and line staff in each hospital. The pre-testing enabled further refinement of the draft instrument, both in terms of substantive content and format. The danger of contagion effect spreading to the formal survey phase was eliminated by conducting the pretest outside New York City.

The final survey instrument incorporated a combination of closed and open-ended items as well as scales and ratings giving the opportunity for the study populations to assess their discharge planning work relative to the new Prospective Payment System impact. Closed-ended items included both those having nominal and Likert-type scaling.

A single instrument was used for both direct service workers and supervisory/administrative personnel. Response categories were sensitive to this and provided 'Not Applicable' type response categories when appropriate.

Study Population

The research strategy was designed to include the universe of discharge planners engaged in discharge planning on medical and surgical units in all New York City acute care hospitals. The goal was to include all coordinators of discharge planning, directors of social work and discharge planning staff in acute care hospitals in the five boroughs of New York City: Manhattan, Bronx, Queens, Brooklyn and Staten Island.

It was estimated by the Discharge Planning Association's Leadership that half of the discharge planners in New York City hospitals are social workers and the other half predominately nurses. It was estimated that approximately 200 personnel in the acute care hospitals in New York City are engaged in discharge planning (Danzig, 1985).

The acute care hospitals of New York City range from very large teaching hospitals, primarily in Manhattan, to small community hospitals in semi-rural areas such as the south shore of Staten Island. Hence, the sample provides a broad range of respondents from hospitals of varying sizes, some of which resemble more suburban, semi-rural institutions.

The rationale for requesting information from all discharge planning coordinators, directors of social work and discharge planners involved in making post-hospital care plans with older adults in this study is clear. There is no standardized model for discharge planning units/departments in acute care hospitals. Approximately half are independent departments headed by a nurse or social worker. While other discharge planning units are a division of social work departments, still others are a division of nursing departments. Regardless of the structure, social workers are involved by a very formalized referral process, by pre-established division of labor guidelines (formal and informal) or as coordinators of discharge planning. The more extensive involvement of social workers as coordinators of discharge planning is unique to New York City. In the rest of the country, this role is primarily fulfilled by nurses (Roberti, 1986).

Data Collection

Two packets were mailed to each acute care hospital subject to the Prospective Payment System (N=77) in Fall, 1986. One packet was sent to the Discharge Planning Coordinator and one to the Director of Social Work. In approximately 15 hospitals, the researcher knew that the director of social work was the designated discharge planning coordinator and for those hospitals, only one packet was mailed. Each packet contained a cover letter to the discharge planning coordinator or director of social work explaining the purpose of the study and asking them to do the following: 1) Complete the questionnaire and return it, and 2) distribute the additional copies enclosed to their discharge planning personnel, targeting the discharge planners assigned to medical-surgical units. The cover letter encouraged anyone to call the researcher if he or she needed extra copies of the questionnaire, although he or she could photocopy additional copies at his or her hospital. If distribution to all staff involved in discharge planning was problematic, it was suggested that a random selection process could be worked out. Finally, the offer was made to come to his or her hospital and administer the questionnaire with a group of staff. Only one hospital chose to have the researcher come for a group administration of the questionnaire.

  The researcher enclosed a number of questionnaires based on her knowledge of hospital bed size and standard staffing patterns. In addition, consultation with key informants from the New York City Discharge Planners Association and Society of Hospital Social Work Directors guided this process. Approximately one dozen hospitals opted to have the researcher send additional questionnaires rather than photocopy it themselves.

Each questionnaire to be distributed to discharge planners had a cover letter addressed, 'Dear Discharge Planner.' It stated the purpose of the study and assured anonymity and confidentiality of individual responses. A stamped, self-addressed envelope was attached to each questionnaire for its return.

Pre-coding the research questionnaire with an individual hospital identification number allowed the researcher to monitor response rates. A two-step follow up method was employed to insure an adequate response rate. First, a telephone call was made after a month of no response, reminding the discharge planning coordinator or director of social work of the study's importance. If there was no response to the telephone call, a letter was mailed approximately three weeks later again reiterating the importance of the study and requesting their participation. Reminders were made by the researcher at two monthly meetings of the New York City Discharge Planners Association. The efforts resulted in a response rate of 75% (N=58 hospitals) with 235 individual discharge planners returning questionnaires.

Protection of Human Subjects

This study was based on individual responses from coordinators of discharge planning and other professional personnel working in discharge planning with the elderly in New York City hospitals. The study surveyed primarily professional staff who could determine for themselves whether to participate in the study. Requests for questionnaire completion were done by mail and only the hospital was coded to insure confidentiality of the respondent while allowing for follow up to insure an adequate response rate. The letter of explanation and request for participation indicated that the study was being carried out to learn about the experiences of discharge planners relative to the elderly and the new prospective payment reimbursement mechanism. It was stated in the cover letter that individual answers would be kept strictly confidential. The interest is in the experience of respondents as a group. Participants could choose not to answer a particular question(s).

Data Analysis

The responses from 75% of the hospitals surveyed, resulted in 235 completed questionnaires.

The first step in the data analysis involved simple descriptive statistics to see important characteristics of the respondents as a whole. The summary statistics were reviewed for differences on measures of central tendency (means and medians) and also on measures of variability (standard deviations and variances). Attention was given to differences of two subsamples;

professional social workers and nurses carrying out discharge planning functions.

The next stage of data analysis involved analyzing differences among the subsample groups as identified above. Since the sampling procedure did not involve the random process, the use of inferential statistics was not applied; rather, this stage relied on a description of the magnitude of relationships that exist in the sample. The most common technique used was the calculation of the size of effect which is analogous to computation of Z scores. Basically, the researcher looked for differences among the subgroups of discharge planners that were meaningful and organizational variables that would help to explain variance.

Chapter 4

PROFILE OF HOSPITAL DISCHARGE PLANNERS

The findings are based on responses received from 58 of the eligible 77 acute care hospitals, which represents a 75.3 percent response rate by facility. A total of 235 individual respondents from the 58 hospitals were received and form the basis for the data analysis. Unfortunately there is no data on exactly how many discharge planners there are in New York City hospitals. Key informants have estimated approximately 200 individuals are involved in discharge planning in New York City hospitals. Based on the number of respondents to this survey, it would appear that 200 is a low estimate.

Hospital Auspice and Bed Size

A summary of the hospitals in New York City and respondents is analyzed by auspice and bed size and reported in Table 4-1.

The auspice of the seventy-seven hospitals shows the majority (67.5%) are voluntary, not-for-profit, while ten (13.0%) are for-profit. The category of public hospitals includes eleven city hospitals, three Veteran's Administration hospitals and one state hospital for a total of fifteen which represents 19.5 percent of the hospitals in New York City. It should be noted that at the time the study was undertaken, the most current listing of hospitals published by the United Hospital Fund of New York was utilized. It listed eighty-three acute care hospitals in the five boroughs of

TABLE 4-1
HOSPITAL CHARACTERISTICS OF RESPONDENTS

Characteristics	Total N	Percent	Respondent N	Percent
NYC Hospitals				
Auspice:				
Public	15	19.5	13	22.4
Not-For-Profit	52	67.5	38	65.5
For-Profit	10	13.0	7	12.1
Total	77	100.0	58	100.0

Bed Size	NYC Hospitals			Hospitals of Respondents		
	Public	Not For Profit	For Profit	Public	Not For Profit	For Profit
0-199	0	7	7	0	5	5
100-399	3	20	3	3	14	2
400-599	4	13	0	3	11	0
600-799	6	8	0	5	6	0
800-999	0	2	0	0	1	0
1000 & Over	2	2	0	2	1	0
Total	15	52	10	13	38	7

Profile of Discharge Planners

New York City. Two hospitals closed during 1986 and four had special exemptions from the Prospective Payment system and were not eligible to participate.

Respondents to the mail questionnaire when analyzed by their hospital's auspice, closely reflect the proportion in existence (Table 4-1). Looking at bed size for all hospitals by auspice and comparing it with the respondent's hospital bed size in this study also confirms a representative respondent pool by bed size.

Profile of Individual Respondents

The profile of the respondent group of discharge planners is based on a number of demographic variables included in the survey instrument. The characteristics of age, sex, race, and education of this group are discussed below and are summarized in Table 4-2.

The age of respondents (discharge planners) ranges from 23 to 69 years of age. The largest grouping by decade cohort is for respondents age 30-39, making up 37 percent. Nothing unusual in the age range or distribution of respondents is observed.

Since social work and nursing are professions entered predominantly by women, it is no surprise that 82 percent of the respondents are female. Eighty-one percent of the respondents are white, 10 percent are black, 6.4 percent are Hispanic and 1.8 are Asian.

Over 80 percent of respondents have a masters degree while 14.1 percent have

TABLE 4-2
Demographic Characteristics of Discharge Planners

Characteristics	Number	Percent
AGE		
20-29	38	17.5
30-39	81	37.3
40-49	56	25.8
50-59	31	14.3
60-69	11	5.1
Total	217	100.0
(Mean Age)	(36.9)	
(Median Age)	(38.0)	
(Mode)	(30)	
(Age Range)	(23-69)	
SEX		
Female	191	82.3
Male	41	17.7
Total	232	100.0
RACE		
White	178	81.3
Black	22	10.0
Hispanic	14	6.4
Asian	4	1.8
Other	1	0.5
Total	219	100.0
HIGHEST EDUCATION		
Less than BA/BS	10	4.2
BS or BA	33	14.1
Masters	188	80.3
Doctorate	3	1.4
Total	234	100.0
PROFESSIONAL DISCIPLINE		
Nursing	28	12.1
Social Work	198	85.3
Other	3	1.3
None	2	1.0
Dual	1	0.3
Total	232	100.0

a bachelors degree, 4.2 percent have less than a bachelor's degree. Only 1 percent did not identify as having a professional discipline. Social work is the predominant profession among respondents. Over eighty-five percent (N=198) of respondents identified social work as their profession while 12 percent identify nursing. This is particularly of interest since in all discussions with key informants in the research development phase, it was estimated that discharge planning was shared about equally between social workers and nurses in acute care hospitals. The remaining 2 percent of respondents claimed another or dual professional discipline. Throughout much of the analysis then, when professional discipline is compared, it was limited to the two groups, social workers and nurses.

Employment Information

Employment status is predominantly full time as reported by 94.4 percent of respondents. While one quarter were employed by the hospital in the past year, almost a third had worked at their current place of employment for two to five years and another 25 percent had been employed by their current hospital for six to thirteen years. See Table 4-3 for a summary of these findings.

The target group was reached, namely, persons performing discharge planning activities on medical surgical divisions of the hospital. While Discharge Planning Coordinators and

TABLE 4-3
EMPLOYMENT INFORMATION OF RESPONDENTS

Characteristics	Number	Percent
EMPLOYMENT STATUS		
Full Time	221	94.4
Part Time	13	5.6
Total	234	100.0
JOB TITLE		
Dir. of Social Work	21	9.4
Ass't. Dir. of Social Work	25	11.2
Social Worker	138	61.8
Social Work Ass't.	13	5.8
Discharge Planning Coord.	11	4.9
Discharge Nurse	11	4.9
Utiliz. Review Personnel	4	1.8
Total	223	100.0
EMPLOYMENT AT CURRENT HOSPITAL		
2-5 Years	74	32.0
6-9 Years	33	14.3
10-13 Years	26	11.3
14-17 Years	26	11.3
18-23 Years	7	3.0
24-30 Years	6	2.6
Total	231	100.0
ENGAGED IN DISCHARGE PLANNING		
1 Year or less	33	14.2
2-5 Years	79	34.1
6-9 Years	43	18.6
10-13 Years	42	18.2
14-17 Years	23	9.9
18-23 Years	7	3.0
24-28 Years	5	2.0
Total	231	100.0

Directors of Social Work were asked to complete the questionnaire _and_ distribute additional copies to discharge planners in their department, analysis by job title reflects the respondents as primarily 'social workers'. The line staff position of social worker accounts for almost 62 percent of respondents. The low number of Discharge Planning Coordinators, almost 5 percent, may be explained by the common practice of the Director of Social Work or the Assistant Director of Social Work having a dual title, which includes Discharge Planning Coordinator. If this explanation is correct, it may support a strong professional identification with social work and a preference for the identification with social work rather than discharge planning per se.

In summary, the respondent populations of discharge planners in acute care hospitals are predominantly white, female, professional social workers who are in their 30's and 40's, employed at their current hospital two or more years, and also engaged in discharge planning activities for two or more years.

Chapter 5

DRGs AND DISCHARGE PLANNERS' ACTIVITIES

This chapter covers the identification of the discharge planning tasks and their frequency. Specific areas in which the Prospective Payment System is associated with changes such as organizational concerns and community resources is presented. Analysis of opinions about DRGs is provided and the tasks pertaining to advising patients of the appeals process concludes the chapter.

(<u>Note</u>: Due to multiple tests of statistical significance, the actual experiment-wise Type 1 error rate would be considerably higher than Alpha=.05 level used in most tests. Hence caution should be exercised in the interpretation but due to the exploratory nature of this study, the researcher has chosen to identify differences which are areas for further research.)

Current Discharge Planning Tasks

Nineteen discharge planning task responsibilities identified in the literature and by key informants provide the basis of an index to determine the frequency with which discharge planners conduct specific activities. Respondents were asked to answer according to the frequency with which they conduct each activity. The category choices ranged from five to one. The response categories were "5" Very Frequently (2-5 times per day), "4" Somewhat Frequently (2-5 times per week), "3" Occasionally

(2-5 times per month), "2" Seldom (2-5 times per year), and "1" Never.

The correlation matrix for the nineteen discharge planning responsibilities revealed inter-item correlations ranging from - 0.14 to 0.88. Generally the higher correlations between discharge planning tasks occur among the direct service type of activities. These items include screening patients for discharge, interviewing elderly patients as to their discharge needs, discussing issues of finance, counseling patients about discharge options, making referrals and counseling patients and/or their significant others. The relationships between the more direct service tasks and the indirect tasks such as participating in research studies, conducting interdisciplinary in-service training programs, supervising own profession's students, teaching other professions' students, and attending continuing education programs tended to be more inversely related.

A principal components factor analysis was done to see whether there existed some underlying pattern of relationship among the nineteen discharge planning tasks. A factor analysis utilizing all respondents (N=235) was executed and five factors with eigenvalues greater than 1 emerged when .3 was used to set the correlation level. Factor 1 only accounted for 28.4 percent of the variance and all five factors combined, only accounted for 61.7 percent of the variance.

The correlation level was then set at .5 with five factors utilizing only social workers (N=198) because the nurse group (N=28) was too small to utilize factor analysis. The total variance explained by five factors with eigenvalues of 1 or more accounted for 61.5 percent. If only three factors are considered, the explained variance drops to 50.0 percent. Therefore it did not seem appropriate to reduce the data because too much information was lost.

A second purpose of utilizing factor analysis was to confirm how variables cluster together in factors. It turned out to be more productive. When a .5 correlation level was utilized, the direct service activities of discharge planning emerged as one factor. This confirmed the grouping of DISAC1 through DISAC8 as discharge planning tasks reflecting direct service activities. DISAC9 was also included because of the nature of the task even though it is not conducted by very many discharge planners (Refer to Table 5-1).

Table 5-1 provides the frequency for the nineteen discharge planning tasks and responsibilities. The table gives a clear picture of 'frequent' activities for DISAC1 through DISAC8 and DISAC10, and then shifts to 'less frequent' for the remaining items. The direct service type of activities are reflected by the variables DISAC1 to DISAC9, covering the areas of screening elderly patients for discharge, interviewing elderly patients to determine service needs, discussing

TABLE 5-1
FREQUENCY OF DISCHARGE PLANNING TASKS

Discharge Activity	N %	Very Frequently	Somewhat Frequently	Frequency of Performance Occasionally	Seldom	Never	Total
DISAC1		158 67.2	55 23.4	14 6.0	5 2.1	3 1.3	235 100.0
DISAC2		146 62.4	61 26.1	17 7.3	7 3.0	3 1.3	234 100.0
DISAC3		122 52.1	78 33.3	22 9.4	8 3.4	4 1.7	234 100.0
DISAC4		147 62.8	60 25.6	17 7.3	7 3.0	3 1.3	234 100.0
DISAC5		141 60.3	67 28.6	19 8.1	6 2.6	1 0.4	234 100.0
DISAC6		103 44.2	87 37.3	26 11.2	10 4.3	7 3.0	233 100.0
DISAC7		72 30.8	107 45.7	35 15.0	13 5.6	7 3.0	234 100.0
DISAC8		86 37.7	76 33.3	36 15.8	15 6.6	15 6.6	228 100.0
DISAC9		10 4.3	7 3.0	21 9.1	41 17.7	152 65.8	231 100.0
DISAC10		139 59.7	55 23.6	18 7.7	9 3.9	12 5.2	233 100.0
DISAC11		8 3.5	13 5.7	42 18.3	61 26.5	106 46.1	230 100.0
DISAC12		15 6.4	41 17.6	116 49.8	44 18.9	17 7.3	233 100.0
DISAC13		4 1.7	3 1.3	15 6.5	115 49.8	94 40.7	231 100.0
DISAC14		4 1.7	11 4.8	46 20.1	82 35.8	86 37.6	229 100.0
DISAC15		11 4.8	23 10.0	12 5.2	25 10.9	159 69.1	230 100.0
DISAC16		1 0.4	12 5.2	21 9.2	55 23.6	144 61.8	233 100.0
DISAC17		2 0.9	9 3.9	133 57.6	63 27.3	24 10.4	231 100.0
DISAC18		5 2.2	19 8.4	84 37.0	68 30.0	51 22.5	227 100.0
DISAC19		49 21.3	91 39.5	64 27.7	21 9.3	5 2.2	230 100.0

DISAC1 = Screen elderly patients
DISAC2 = Interview elderly patients' service needs
DISAC3 = Discuss issues of finances
DISAC4 = Counsel patients about discharge options
DISAC5 = Make referrals on patients' behalf
DISAC6 = Provide counseling to patient
DISAC7 = Provide counseling to patient's family
DISAC8 = Casefinding in the hospital
DISAC9 = Pre-admission assessments
DISAC10 = Routine recordkeeping
DISAC11 = Community education/elderly
DISAC12 = Explore new services
DISAC13 = Participate research
DISAC14 = Conduct interdisc. in-service
DISAC15 = Supervise "own" prof. students
DISAC16 = Teach "other" prof. students
DISAC17 = Attend continuing education
DISAC18 = Inform patients of Appeals
DISAC19 = Advocate/service providers

Activities

finances, counseling patients and their families about discharge arrangement options, psychosocial counseling, casefinding in the hospital and preadmission screening.

The 'Very Frequently' and 'Somewhat Frequently' response categories reflect a range of 91 percent to 71.0 percent of activities. The highest frequency among all activities is 'screening elderly patients needs for discharge' which accounts for 67 percent of the 'Very Frequently' responses, and 90 percent when the 'Somewhat Frequently' response category is included.

DISAC9 refers to the frequency of doing pre-admission assessments among elective medical-surgical patients and the majority, 66 percent, reported 'Never". The discharge planning literature had projected an increase in this activity in a cost-containment climate which is not supported by these data. It may be too soon to see this type of activity change within this first year of implementation of the Prospective Payment System in New York. This particular variable deserves further subsequent consideration.

DISAC10 through DISAC19 reflect indirect types of discharge planning activities. They included routine recordkeeping, community education with older adults, exploring new services, participating in research, conducting inservice education, supervising one's own and other professional students, attending continuing education, informing patients of appeals, and advocating with service providers. With the exception of routine recordkeeping (DISAC10) and advocacy with service providers (DISAC19) which account for 60 percent and 21 percent respectively, of the 'very frequently' response choice, the frequency of the more indirect discharge planning activities moves across the table to the less frequent performance side as reflected in the bottom half of Table 5-1.

A comparison of how nurses and social workers differ in reporting the frequency of performing these nineteen discharge planning tasks is provided in Table 5-2. Four discharge planning tasks were found to differ between nurses and social workers at a statistically significant level. The first refers to the discharge planning task of discussing with a patient issues of finance (DISAC3). Social workers were more frequently engaged in this task than nurses as reflected by the T-value ($t=-2.33$; $p<0.02$). The second activity is in the provision of psychosocial counseling to patients (DISAC6); nurses are less frequently engaged in this discharge planning task than social workers ($t=-4.38$; $p=0.000$). This same trend is observed for the discharge activity of providing psychosocial counseling to a patient's family (DISAC7). Nurses are less frequently involved in this task relative to discharge planning than social workers ($t=-3.84$; $p<0.001$).

The fourth and final task which

TABLE 5-2
DISCHARGE PLANNING TASKS
BY RESPONDENT TYPE

Characteristic	Nurse Mean	S.D.	Social Work Mean	S.D.	T-Value (2-tail Prob) Mean	S.D.
DISAC 1	4.54	0.88	4.52	0.81	0.009	0.930
2	4.07	1.18	4.49	0.80	-1.82	0.078
3	3.79	1.32	4.38	0.82	-2.33	0.027**
4	4.04	1.29	4.51	0.77	-1.89	0.069
5	4.25	1.01	4.48	0.76	-1.15	0.259
6	3.14	1.38	4.31	0.83	-4.38	0.000**
7	3.11	1.34	4.11	0.83	-3.84	0.001**
8	4.00	1.33	3.86	1.17	0.51	0.612
9	1.78	1.19	1.60	1.05	0.75	0.458
10	4.36	1.03	4.29	1.11	0.34	0.735
11	1.63	1.01	2.00	1.11	-1.77	0.085
12	2.96	1.14	2.98	0.94	-0.09	0.928
13	1.93	1.11	1.74	0.73	0.85	0.400
14	2.21	1.07	1.94	0.92	1.28	0.209
15	1.50	0.96	1.77	1.27	-1.31	0.197
16	1.61	0.92	1.61	0.90	0.00	1.000
17	2.70	0.61	2.57	0.78	1.00	0.325
18	2.04	1.17	2.43	0.96	-1.72	0.095
19	2.96	1.29	3.71	1.04	-2.93	0.006**

DISAC 1 = Screen Elderly Patients
DISAC 2 = Interview for Discharge Needs
DISAC 3 = Discuss Issues of Finance
DISAC 4 = Counsel on Discharge Options
DISAC 5 = Make Referrals for Service Needs
DISAC 6 = Counsel Patient
DISAC 7 = Counsel Family
DISAC 8 = Casefind in Hospital
DISAC 9 = Pre-Admit Screen
DISAC 10 = Record Keeping
DISAC 11 = Conduct Community Education
DISAC 12 = Explore New Services
DISAC 13 = Participate in Research
DISAC 14 = Conduct Interdisciplinary Training
DISAC 15 = Supervise (own profession's) Students
DISAC 16 = Teach Other Profession's Students
DISAC 17 = Attend Continuing Education
DISAC 18 = Inform Patients of Appeals
DISAC 19 = Advocate for Patients with Service Providers

**Statistical Significance

reflected a statistically significant difference between nurses and social workers refers to advocacy for patients with service providers (DISAC19). Social workers report being more frequently involved in this discharge planning task than were nurses (t=-2.93; p<0.006).

To complete the assessment of the current tasks of discharge planning, five more variables were analyzed. The first item inquired as to the average weekly size of a discharge planning caseload of older adults (defined as patients who are age 65 and over). The average number of patients seen per week ranged from 1 to 250 with 10 percent of respondents reporting that they do not see patients. There are three clusters of patients representing the average number of patients seen. The first group were 'less than 20 per week', the next group was '20 to 30 per week' and the last group was 'over 30' per week. Seventy-five percent of the average weekly caseloads seen for discharge planning are elderly. Table 5-3 portrays the average weekly caseload and its percentage of elderly as reported by respondents.

The high percentage of elderly persons reported by respondents seen per week for discharge planning purposes is important for two reasons. First, it reflects the growing number of older adults in the population and that on the national average, 30 percent of all hospital beds are occupied by older adults. Secondly, it validated that the

TABLE 5-3
AVERAGE WEEKLY CASELOAD AND PROPORTION ELDERLY

Characteristic	Number	Percent
Average Number Patients Seen per Weekly Discharge		
1-19	65	31.6
20-29	70	34.0
30-39	39	18.9
40-59	21	10.2
60 & Over	11	5.3
TOTAL	206	100.0
Elderly as Percentage of Caseload		
1-25 Percent	14	6.6
26-50 Percent	36	17.9
51-75 Percent	50	24.6
76-100 Percent	103	50.9
TOTAL	203	100.0

80 *Prospective Payments and Discharge Planning*

target respondent group for this study, discharge planners who serve the elderly on medical-surgical units, participated.

Two items asked respondents about their ability to follow up with patients who were discharged and the service providers who gave care to the discharged patients. Frequency data are reported by respondent type, nurses and social workers, on follow-up in Table 5-4. It shows nurses following up with discharged elderly 'all the time' with a 36 percent frequency. Social workers report follow up with discharged patients 'all the time' with 22 percent frequency. When the 'all the time' and 'sometimes' category are combined, the frequency for nurses is 64 percent and 62 percent for social workers. The difference of the means for the two respondent groups is not statistically significant.

The importance of high-risk screening for all patients admitted to an acute care hospital has been well documented in the literature. Data were gathered from respondents as to which high risk screening criteria they utilize. Table 5-5 reports these data for nurse and social worker respondents. Age and diagnosis are the most frequently reported criteria. These two criteria are utilized in 98 percent of the hospitals. The descending order in frequency for high risk criteria are as follows: living arrangements, functional status, family support, post hospital

TABLE 5-4
FOLLOW-UP FREQUENCY POST DISCHARGE
BY NURSES AND SOCIAL WORKERS

Characteristic	"YES" All The Time (1)	Some- times (2)	Rarely (3)	No (4)	Do Not Know (5)	Total (N)
A. Follow-Up with Patients						
NURSES	35.7%	28.6%	25.0%	7.1%	3.6%	27
SOCIAL WORKERS	22.4	49.2	16.6	10.7	1.0	116
B. Follow-Up with Providers						
NURSES	46.4	17.9	21.4	7.1	7.1	28
SOCIAL WORKERS	24.9	45.7	15.7	8.6	3.6	194

TABLE 5-5
HIGH RISK SCREEN CRITERIA
BY RESPONDENT TYPE

Characteristic	Nurse		Social Work		T-VALUE (2 Tail Prob)	
	Mean	S.D.	Mean	S.D.	Mean	S.D.
HIGH RISK SCREEN CRITERIA						
a) Age	1.07	0.26	1.02	0.12	1.11	0.275
b) Sex	1.70	0.47	1.81	0.47	-1.14	0.263
c) Family Support	1.21	0.42	1.28	0.45	-0.81	0.423
d) Diagnosis	1.07	0.26	1.02	0.12	1.11	0.275
e) Financial Information	1.29	0.46	1.37	0.48	-0.91	0.368
f) Living Arrangements	1.21	0.42	1.17	0.38	0.53	0.600
g) Functional Status	1.43	0.50	1.22	0.41	2.14	0.040**
h) Post Hospital Needs	1.43	0.50	1.31	0.47	1.15	0.259

t = Theoretical Index Item Range: 1-2; Where 1 = YES and 2 = NO. Thus a lower score reflects a more prevalent use of the variable in high risk screening criteria.

**Statistically Significant

needs, financial information, and sex of patients.

Correlation by respondent type for the high risk screen components shows only one that is statistically significant in its difference between social workers and nurses. Social workers report a higher frequency of utilization of a patient's functional status as a high risk screen criteria than nurses ($t=2.14$; $p<0.040$). This presents an unanticipated result.

The responsibility for conducting high risk screening is most frequently attributed to social work departmental staff (89.7%); followed by utilization review staff (46.2%); followed by discharge planning staff (39.3%). The lower reporting of discharge planning staff having responsibility for high risk screening is surprising. However, it most likely reflects the organizational prevalence for discharge planning units/divisions to be a part of social work departments in this study population of New York City hospitals.

Time Allocation on Discharge Tasks

This area of inquiry assessed how the time spent on various discharge planning task responsibilities may have changed due to the impact of the Prospective Payment System (DRG) legislation. The inquiry also included several other items regarding potential areas of change in the ways discharge planning is conducted with the elderly such as frequency of interdisciplinary meeting, referrals, case management need, and Resource Utilization Groupings (RUGs) for nursing home admissions.

An underlying thesis shaping this study was the belief that the Prospective Payment System of reimbursement for hospital care would have an impact on discharge planning tasks resulting from the increased pressure to discharge elderly patients as soon as possible to conserve costs. It was also hypothesized that while there is no clear role delineation between social workers and nurses, they may respond differently to the discharge planning pressures created by DRGs.

The nineteen discharge planning tasks (direct and indirect) reported in the previous section (DISAC1 through DSISAC19) were repeated in the questionnaire and respondents asked to indicate if the time spent on each task responsibility had increased, decreased or not changed since DRGs went into effect. Items in this measure were scored on a five point scale. Time spent on each task was scored: 5=markedly increased, 4=increased, 3=no change, 2=decreased, and 1=markedly decreased. The limitation of this scale is that it requires the respondent to retrospectively compare how time was spent on discharge tasks prior to DRG inauguration. the ideal alternative would have been pre-DRG data collection as a baseline, however, this was not feasible.

DRGs and Discharge Planners Activities

In reviewing the correlation matrix for time spent on discharge tasks affected by DRGs, the inter-item correlations ranged from -.23 to .89. The pattern of time spent on the nineteen items is similar to the frequency of their performance previously discussed.

Utilizing the grouping of items from the initial confirmatory factor analysis, the time spent on direct service discharge tasks (DISTM1 through DISTM9) and indirect tasks (DISTM10 through DISTM19) are compared by the two respondent group types, nurses and social workers. The data are summarized in Table 5-6.

The highest increase in time spent on tasks related to discharge planning for nurses is DISTM10, which refers to recordkeeping (Mean-4.07). The highest increase among social workers is DISTM1 which refers to screening elderly patients for discharge (mean=3.99).

The overall trend for both social workers and nurses in reporting how their time is spent on discharge planning tasks since DRGs went into effect is primarily one of increased time spent on the direct service types of tasks and two indirect service tasks which consist of informing patients of appeals (DISTM18) and advocating with service providers (DISTM19) respectively. With these two exceptions, the indirect type of discharge planning tasks tended to reflect decreased time spent for both nurses and social workers on the items of supervision of students (respondent's own profession), and teaching (other

TABLE 5-6
TIME SPENT ON DISCHARGE PLANNING TASKS AFFECTED BY DRG'S RESPONDENT TYPE

Characteristic:	Nurse		Social Work		F-Value (2 tail Prob)	
	Mean	S.D.	Mean	S.D.	Mean	S.D.
DISTM 1	4.04	0.71	3.99	0.90	0.31	0.755
2	4.00	0.73	3.91	0.80	0.57	0.573
3	3.85	0.86	3.85	0.85	0.01	0.994
4	3.96	0.76	3.95	0.88	0.06	0.953
5	4.04	0.71	3.96	0.84	0.53	0.602
6	3.52	0.80	3.15	0.97	2.19	0.035**
7	3.44	0.75	3.22	0.99	1.38	0.177
8	3.74	0.90	3.37	1.03	1.96	0.057**
9	3.08	0.85	2.93	0.82	0.86	0.398
10	4.07	0.78	3.71	0.92	2.21	0.033**
11	2.96	0.44	2.96	0.71	0.04	0.964
12	3.52	0.85	3.44	0.83	0.45	0.658
13	3.00	0.72	2.83	0.65	1.18	0.248
14	3.14	0.59	2.99	0.75	1.19	0.240
15	2.89	0.58	2.82	0.70	0.58	0.564
16	2.93	0.60	2.85	0.67	0.64	0.525
17	3.21	0.42	2.97	0.73	2.53	0.014**
18	3.28	0.74	3.29	0.62	-0.03	0.974
19	3.29	1.15	3.56	0.92	-1.19	0.243

t Scale Metrics: 1-5: Where 1 = Markedly Decreased; 2 = Decreased; 3 = No Change; 4 = Increased; 5 = Markedly Increased. Potential score range: 19-95

DISTM 1 = Screen Elderly Patients
DISTM 2 = Interview for Discharge Needs
DISTM 3 = Discuss Issues of Finance
DISTM 4 = Counsel Patients on Discharge Options
DISTM 5 = Make Referrals for Service Needs
DISTM 6 = Counsel Patient
DISTM 7 = Counsel Family
DISTM 8 = Casefind in Hospital
DISTM 9 = Pre-Admit Screen
DISTM 10 = Record Keeping
DISTM 11 = Conduct Community Education
DISTM 12 = Explore New Services
DISTM 13 = Participate in Research
DISTM 14 = Conduct Interdisciplinary Training
DISTM 15 = Supervise (own profession's) Students
DISTM 16 = Teach Other Profession's Students
DISTM 17 = Attend Continuing Education
DISTM 18 = Inform Patients of Appeals Process
DISTM 19 = Advocate With Service Providers

**Statistically Significant

professions') students. A decrease in time spent among social work respondents only is documented in tasks of conducting community education programs, participating in research, and attending continuing education programs.

There are four discharge planning tasks where social workers and nurses differ on how much time spent has changed due to DRGs. The first discharge planning task where a statistically significant difference is observed is in providing psychosocial counseling to patients (DISTM6). Nurses do report time spent on this task as increased due to DRGs in greater proportion than social workers (t=2.19; p<0.035). The same trend is also observed in time spent on casefinding in the hospital (DISTM8), nurses report a larger increase than social workers (t=1.96; p<0.057).

The most marked increase in time spent on discharge planning tasks due to DRGs among nurses was routine recordkeeping (DISTM10). It was statistically significantly different from social workers at the .05 level (t=2.21; p<0.033). The final area of statistical significance among the nineteen items on how time spent on discharge planning tasks has changed was attending continuing education programs (DISTM17). Nurses reported more of an increase in the time spent attending programs than social workers (t=2.53; p<0.014).

Other than the variable of professional discipline, respondent's employment tenure and years in discharge planning work, were not correlated with how time spent on discharge planning tasks has changed due to DRGs. The two organizational variables of auspice and bed size of the hospital were not associated with time spent on discharge tasks with one exception. The task of interviewing elderly patients as to service needs for discharge was statistically significant with bed size of hospitals (x^2 =21.2; p<0.047). The large hospitals of 600 and over beds were more likely to report 'markedly increased' time spent on the area, interviewing elderly patients for determination of services need.

In addition to the nineteen item scale of discharge planning tasks and responsibilities, five additional areas of potential DRG-induced change were examined. The areas of: 1) inpatient and outpatient populations; 2) formal and informal meetings for discharge planning purposes; 3) referral requirements; 4) case management service need; and 5) Resource Utilization Groupings (RUGS) effect on nursing home admissions. Findings in each area follow.

Inpatient and Outpatient Populations

Changes in both the inpatient and outpatient populations seen for discharge planning were queried. The change in the inpatient population seen for discharge planning was perceived very differently by nurses than by social workers. While

55 percent of social workers reported an increase in the inpatient population seen for discharge planning, only 25 percent of nurses reported similarly. Forty-six percent of the nurse respondents were unaware of changes in the inpatient population seen for discharge planning while only 13 percent of social workers replied similarly. One interpretation suggests that social workers are more aware of this increase as a consequence of what they perceive as role restrictions brought about by increased discharge caseloads. Nurse, on the other hand, may have left their bedside role precisely to do discharge planning. For nurses it is a new job, for social workers a narrowing of focus.

Upon further investigation of changes in the inpatient populations seen for discharge planning, an interesting finding emerged among respondents based on their length of employment. Discharge planners employed eleven years or more at their current hospital reported no increase in the inpatient population seen for discharge planning which they attribute to PPS/DRG. Perhaps these more experienced workers viewed DRGs as just another cyclical change in the hospitals operation. Another interpretation may be that given the demographic bulge of older adult cohorts, the inpatient population seen for discharge planning, has and will continue to increase naturally. As more elderly live longer, there will be more need for discharge planning which has nothing to do with DRGs specifically. Auspice and bedsize of the hospital also have not significantly affected the perception of inpatient population change by discharge planners.

Interdisciplinary Team Meetings

Discharge planners responding to the survey were asked to assess the change in frequency, if any, of interdisciplinary team meetings for purposes related to discharge planning. The data for utilization of formal interdisciplinary team meetings and the change in frequency, if any, attributable to DRGs showed that 72 percent of all respondents report 'no change' due to DRGs. While 17 percent of discharge planners reported more frequent interdisciplinary team meetings, 3 percent reported 'less frequent' team meetings. It appears that formal team meetings for purposes of discharge planning have not been affected by DRGs.
Informal meetings for discharge planning purposes showed a large increase among all discharge planners. The majority of respondents, (72%) regardless of professional discipline, report an increase in informal meetings for discharge planning purposes since DRGs went into effect. Under 2 percent report less frequency for informal team meetings, 22 percent report no change and 4 percent report they do not know. These data do support an area of change attributable to DRGs namely, frequency of

Activities

informal meetings for purposes of discharge planning.

Referral Requirements

Initially in medical social work practice, a referral from a patient's physician was required before a social worker could see a patient. The current practice was an area of inquiry of this study.

The freedom to see any patient in the acute care hospital setting has now become an almost universally accepted practice. Over 95 percent of all respondents, regardless of discipline, were able to see any patient without a referral. Among the 5 percent of discharge planners who reported they must have a referral, eight were social workers and two were nurses. Clearly, the ability to identify any patient who may need discharge planning services and to intervene is common practice. This may be viewed as more independent, professional practice for discharge planners who are working in a host organization such as a hospital.

Case Management Service Needs

One area of inquiry focused on case management service need. It was an outgrowth of the claim that since patients are being discharged 'quicker and sicker' from hospitals, there would be a greater need for case managers to orchestrate the maze of services on behalf of elderly patients. One study completed for the National Association of Area Agencies on Aging documented the impact which DRGs are having on community based services (Harlow and Wilson, 1985). It indicated that case management service units increased 365 percent after DRG implementation in their study population which were agencies receiving Older American Act funds for case management services. The 365 percent increase in case management services is in contrast to the next highest category, in-home skilled nursing, which showed a 196 percent increase (Harlow and Wilson, 1985, p.6). The rationale provided in their study was that since patients are being discharged 'quicker and sicker', there is greater need to manage the service maze on behalf of clients discharged back to the community.

Findings of this study supported the conclusions of Harlow and Wilson. Seventy-five percent of all respondents report in fact, that the need for case management services since DRGs went into effect has increased. A mere 11 percent reported a decrease, 13 percent reported no change and 11 percent reported they did not know if case management needs had increased since DRGs went into effect. There were basically no differences between nurses and social workers in their perception of the increased need for case management services since DRGs.

In anticipation of this finding that case management service needs had increased since DRGs went into effect, it was of interest to inquire to whom discharge planners refer patients for case management. Seven referral options were provided namely, a) social workers in my hospital, b) Visiting Nurse Service, c) Human Resource Administration home care programs, d) NYC Department for the Aging home care programs, e) case managers within (own) hospitals' home health care program, f) private geriatric practitioners, g) for-profit home health care agency and h) with an 'other' category and scaled by frequency. The frequency scale range was: 1=never, 2=rarely, 3=sometimes, and 4=most often. Since only 16 responses (less than 10%) were reported for 'other,' this response category was dropped. The potential score range was 7 (never use referral source) to 28 (most often use referral source). Inter-item correlations ranged from -.13 to .37 and did not reveal very strong correlations among the seven referral sources for case management services.

Table 5-7 documents where hospital discharge planners, both social workers and nurses, referred patients who need case management services. Only one referral source for case management showed a statistically significant difference (p<.001) between nurses and social workers. Referral to private geriatric practitioners (REFER6) was less likely to be utilized by nurses than social workers.

If the referral sources were ranked according to the mean scores from the most frequent to the least frequent,

TABLE 5-7
CASE MANAGEMENT REFERRAL SOURCE BY RESPONDENT TYPE

Referral Source	Nurse (N=28)		Social Work (N=198)		T-VALUE 2-Tail Prob.	
	Mean	S.D.	Mean	S.D.		
REFER. 1	3.12	1.07	2.89	1.47	0.97	0.341
REFER. 2	3.29	0.85	3.15	1.09	0.78	0.442
REFER. 3	2.75	1.11	2.86	1.20	-0.48	0.634
REFER. 4	1.50	1.07	1.69	1.14	-0.88	0.385
REFER. 5	1.75	1.62	1.96	1.64	-0.64	0.527
REFER. 6	0.79	0.50	1.17	0.88	-3.36	0.001**
REFER. 7	2.00	1.16	2.25	1.14	-1.06	0.295

Scale Metrics: 1-4: Where 1 = Never; 2 = Rarely; 3 = Sometimes 4 = Most Often

REFER 1 = Social Worker in My Hospital
REFER 2 = Visiting Nurse Associate
REFER 3 = HRA Home Care Program
REFER 4 = DFTA Home Care Programs
REFER 5 = My Hospital's Home Care
REFER 6 = Private Geriatric Practitioner
REFER 7 = For-Profit Home Health Care Agency

**Statistically Significant

social workers and nurses are in agreement. The most frequent referral source for case management services was the Visiting Nurse Service with the mean score for nurses being 3.29 and the mean score for social workers being 3.15.

It is interesting to note that while the Visiting Nurse Service was identified as the principal agency used for referral, they have limited capability for accepting a sliding fee scale and rely heavily on Medicare reimbursement. Medicare reimbursement promotes a medical model of care which stresses acute care needs, not chronic care. In the late summer of 1986, Visiting Nurse Service of Manhattan terminated all of its social workers as a result of lost revenues and tightened eligibility for services under Medicare reimbursement. It seemed a tragedy that Visiting Nursing Service was seen as the primary referral source for case management services when in fact it had curtailed providing services to patients not needing all but the most 'skilled' care under Medicare's definition. What happened to the case management service need is an area requiring further study.

The second most frequent referral source for case management services was each respondent's 'own hospital social workers.' The data showed that hospital social workers do not routinely follow up with discharge patients or with their arranged service providers, a contradictory finding since follow up tasks are crucial to case management.

The remaining referral sources are noted in Table 5-7.

Resource Utilization Groupings (RUGs)

Concurrent with the implementation of the Prospective Payment System for Medicare-eligible hospital patients, New York State instituted a prospective form of Medicaid reimbursement to nursing homes. As of January 1986, nursing homes were paid for patients' care based on a case-mix basis with the more skilled level of care receiving a higher reimbursement than more chronic, less-skilled care.

The anticipated finding was that nursing homes would prefer to admit the more frail patients who require more highly skilled care. This would be a direct reversal of the types of patients preferred by nursing homes for admission prior to the implementation of RUGs. Nursing homes would obviously want to maximize their reimbursement rate and would change their priority for admission to patients with more skilled-care needs. Almost three quarters (74%) of all respondents verified that nursing homes prefer patients requiring more skilled care since the implementation of RUGs. A very modest 5 percent felt that nursing homes prefer the patient requiring less skilled-care, only 2.6 percent perceived 'no change' in the type of patients nursing homes are admitting, while 17.9 percent are 'not sure'.

Activities

When the data were analyzed by respondent type, nurses were almost unanimously (93%) of the opinion that RUGs is responsible for nursing home preference for admission of the more skilled-level type of patient. Social workers supported the statement that RUGs had made an impact on nursing homes' preference for admitting more skilled-need patients among 72 percent of respondents. Almost twenty percent reported 'not knowing' if RUGs had influenced nursing home admissions. The difference between nurses and social workers' responses to this question was statistically significant ($t=-2.87$; $p<0.01$).

To summarize, the attribution of time spent on various discharge tasks significantly changed due to DRGs. The additional five areas of inquiry documented change in four areas. First, an increase in both inpatient and outpatient populations seen for discharge planning services; second, an increase in informal interdisciplinary team meetings for the purpose of discharge planning although no increase in the formal interdisciplinary team meetings was reported; third, case management service-needs had greatly increased since DRGs went into effect; fourth, the type of patients which nursing homes accept for admission has altered due to another form of prospective payment, Resource Utilization Groupings (RUGs).

Discharge Planner Opinions

An adaptation of a DRG Opinion scale, based on the results of a study conducted in central Illinois by Michael Patchner and Shirley Wattenberg (1985), was utilized. Their study assessed the anticipated impact of DRGs, just prior to their implementation in 1984, on Illinois hospital social service departments. A survey questionnaire was mailed to 22 directors of social work who were members of the Central Illinois Society of Hospital Social Work Directors. Since the Patchner and Wattenberg scale asked respondents to project how DRGs will affect their role, work, service organization and delivery, the scale utilized in the present study kept nine similar items and added four additional ones.

Table 5-8 presents the thirteen item DRG opinion scale by respondent type (social workers and nurses). It documents that discharge planners do perceive changes attributable to DRGs in the areas of role enhancement, hospital service delivery, coordination of patient care, and their discharge planning work. Regarding the first two opinion statements which ask respondents if DRGs will enhance coordination of patient care (DRGOP1) and if DRGs will generally make the hospital more efficient (DRGOP2P, nurses and social workers report disagreement. They do not feel DRGs will enhance coordination of patient care or

DRGs and Discharge Planners Activities

TABLE 5-8
DRG OPINIONS BY RESPONDENT TYPE

Category	Nurse Mean	S.D.	Social Work Mean	S.D.	t-Value (2-tail Prob) T-Val.	2-Tail
DRGOP 1	3.37	1.08	3.63	0.96	-1.18	0.246
DRGOP 2	3.07	1.21	3.48	1.01	-1.67	0.105
DRGOP 3	2.56	1.28	3.07	1.18	-1.98	0.056
DRGOP 4	2.96	1.22	3.10	1.16	-0.55	0.584
DRGOP 5	2.52	1.16	3.04	1.13	-2.21	0.034*
DRGOP 6	2.21	1.03	2.06	1.01	0.73	0.467
DRGOP 7	2.71	1.18	2.35	1.07	1.53	0.134
DRGOP 8	2.89	1.20	3.45	0.98	-2.37	0.024*
DRGOP 9	3.54	1.07	3.73	0.96	-0.92	0.364
DRGOP 10	2.67	1.07	2.26	1.11	1.85	0.073
DRGOP 11	3.68	0.95	4.07	0.91	-2.04	0.049*
DRGOP 12	2.46	1.23	2.49	1.21	-0.11	0.911
DRGOP 13	1.89	0.89	2.59	1.07	-3.73	0.001*

DRGOP 1 = Enhance Coordination of Patient Care
DRGOP 2 = Make Hospital More Efficient
DRGOP 3 = Strengthen Role on Health Team
DRGOP 4 = Enhance Role Among Physicians
DRGOP 5 = Enhance Role Non-Physicians
DRGOP 6 = Increase Service/Decreased Resources
DRGOP 7 = Higher Priority to Medicare Patients
DRGOP 8 = Enhanced Relationship of Hospital and Community
DRGOP 9 = Favorably Effect Efficiency
DRGOP 10 = Some Patients Will Get Less Care
DRGOP 11 = Better to Discharge Patients Quicker
DRGOP 12 = Should Improve Severity of Illness
DRGOP 13 = Eventually All Patients Covered by PPS

t Scale Metrics: 1 = Strongly Agree; 2 = Agree; 3 = Remain Neutral;
    4 = Disagree; 5 = Strongly Disagree

*Statistically Significant

make the hospital more efficient.

The next three opinion statements refer to areas of role enhancement, first among the health care team (DRGOP3), then among physicians (DRGOP4), and then among hospital personnel who are not physicians (DRGOP5). The mean rating scores for nurses range from 2.52 to 2.96 which indicates agreement with these statements that DRGs have enhanced their role among the three groups identified. Social workers were more negative, although closer to remaining neutral. The mean scores for social workers on the three opinion statements regarding their role enhancement ranged from 3.04 to 3.10. One area of role enhancement, that being among physicians, was statistically significant in its mean difference between social workers and nurses ($t=-2.21$; $p<0.034$).

"DRG's can cause hospital administration to pressure for increased services with fewer resources (DRGOP6)" and "discharge planners are experiencing pressure to give higher priority to Medicare eligible patients because of DRGs (DRGOP7)" are two opinion statements where social workers and nurses show agreement. Both respondent groups agree with these statements. Both opinion statements have role-stressing implications.

"DRGs will enhance the relationship between the hospital and community agency" (DRGOP8), produced statistically significant differences between nurse and social work respondents (t=-2.37; p<0.024). Nurses agreed with this statement while social workers disagreed.

Inquiry as to whether DRGs will favorably affect efficiency in delivery of health care (DRGOP9), and the statement that some patients in my hospital will receive less care because of DRGs, (DRGOP10), finds social workers and nurses in agreement. Regarding the favorable effect on efficiency in delivery of health care, both respondent groups disagreed. As for the statement that some patients will receive less care, both groups of respondents agree. "It is better that patients are being discharged quicker and sicker, due to DRGs" (DRGOP11), found both nurses and social workers disagreeing with the statement. The degree of difference between their mean scores was statistically significant at the level of .05 (t=-2.04; p<0.049).

Inquiry among respondents as to improving the severity-of-illness index to better reflect multiple conditions (DRGOP12), resulted in mutual agreement with this statement by nurses and social workers. The last opinion statement asked whether respondents feel that eventually, patients of all ages will be reimbursed through a Prospective Payment System. Nurses and social workers both agreed with this statement. Nurses more strongly agreed than social work respondents at a statistically significant level (t=-3.73; p<0.001).

In addition to professional discipline, a respondent's job title was

102 Prospective Payments and Discharge Planning

explored to see if it would have some predictor capability in his or her opinions about DRGs. Due to the broad range of job titles of respondents, it was not possible to conduct a meaningful chi-square statistic to correlate the two variables.

One area of interest was whether the auspice of a hospital had any impact on how discharge planners perceive DRGs. The thirteen items of the DRG opinion scale were correlated with the auspice of respondents' hospitals. Regarding auspice, the overall question was whether respondents from the three types (groups) of hospitals, the public, the not-for-profit, and the for-profit, were the same in their opinions about DRGs. The answer was yes except for two opinion items.

Post-hoc comparisons among the three groups was conducted using the Student-Newman-Keuls Procedure with Alpha, the probability of Type 1 error, set at .05. The ranges for the .05 level are 2.81 to 3.34.

The DRGOP5 item asked respondents if DRGs will enhance their role among hospital (non-physician) personnel. As Table 5-9 shows, there was a statistically significant difference between Group 1, the public hospitals and Group 2, the not-for-profit hospitals ($F=4.22$; $p<.0158$). The public hospital respondents were more negative in their response than the not-for-profit hospital respondents.

TABLE 5-9
DRG OPINIONS BY AUSPICE OF HOSPITAL

DRG Opinion 5^t = DRGs will enhance my role among hospital personnel (non-physician)

ANALYSIS OF VARIANCE

SOURCE	D.F.	SUM OF SQUARES	MEAN SQUARES	F RATIO	F PROBABILITY
Between Group	2	10.56	5.28	4.22	0.00158**
With Group	228	285.16	1.25		
Total	230	295.72			

GROUP/AUSPICE	COUNT	MEAN	S.D.
1 = Public	65	3.28	1.21
2 = Not for Profit	155	2.98	1.10
3 = For Profit	11	2.45	0.82

t-Scale Metrics: 1-5 where: 1 = Strongly Agree; 2 = Agree; 3 = Remain Neutral; 4 = Disagree; 5 = Strongly Disagree

**Statistically Significant

Table 5-10 shows the second DRG opinion in which auspice produced a difference between groups. DRGOP8 asked whether DRGs will enhance the relationship between the hospital and community agencies. Differences at the P<.05 level of significance occurred between Group 3, the for-profit hospitals and Groups 2 and 1, the not-for-profit and public hospitals respondents respectively. The for-profit hospital respondents were more inclined to agree with the statement that DRGs will enhance the relationship between the hospital and community than are the not-for-profit and public hospitals. The public hospitals were least favorably inclined to rate this statement affirmatively (F=3.43; P<.034). Often public hospitals are viewed as the place of last resort, no one can be turned away. This may have an impact on the opinion statement that DRGs were not viewed to enhance the relationship between the hospital and community agencies.

A respondent's length of employment at the hospital and the years of experience in discharge planning work were significantly correlated with one DRG opinion scale item, namely, the opinion that some patients will receive less care. When correlated with years of employment, those discharge planners who had been employed the least amount of time were more likely to agree with this statement (x^2 =33.9; p<0.0007). This same trend was observed for the

TABLE 5-10
DRG OPINION BY AUSPICE OF HOSPITAL

DRG Opinion 8^t = DRG's will enhance the relationship between the hospital and community aging.

ANALYSIS OF VARIANCE

SOURCE	D.F	SUM OF SQUARES	MEAN SQUARES	F RATIO	F PROBABILITY
Between Group	2	7.13	3.57	3.43	0.340**
Within Group	229	237.96	1.04		
Total	231	245.09			

GROUP/AUSPICE	MEAN	S.D.
1 = Public	3.57	1.03
2 = Not for Profit	3.36	0.97
3 = For Profit	2.75	1.48

t-Scale Metrics: 1-5 where: 1 = Strongly Agree; 2 = Agree; 3 = Remain Neutral; 4 = Disagree; 5 = Strongly Disagree

**Statistically Significant

respondent's years of discharge planning experience. The less experienced discharge planners were more likely to respond that some patients will get less care because of DRGs (x^2 =21.1; p<0.0487).

Advising Patients About Appeals

The new Prospective Payment System legislation brought with it increased monitoring of utilization of hospital resources and a requirement that all patients be advised of their rights to appeal discharge decisions. In New York State patients must be given written information about their right to appeal. The discharge planner is a key health care team professional who is very likely to be confronted by the patient and his/her family network about disagreements concerning the date of discharge.

Four specific items in the questionnaire relate to the appeal mechanism and the general process of giving information about DRGs to consumers. The first item refers to one of the nineteen items on the discharge planning task responsibilities index. In looking once again at Table 5-1, the frequencies for all respondents reveals that 'informing patients about the appeals mechanism' (DISAC18) is not very frequent. In combining the 'very frequently' and 'somewhat frequently' response choices, only 24 respondents'

DRGs and Discharge Planners Activities

(10.6%) accounts for these two frequencies.

The changes in time spent on the specific task of informing patients of the appeal mechanisms was identified by the index of time spent on discharge planning tasks as affected by DRGs (DISTM18); refer back to Table 5-6. It showed an increase in time spent for both nurses and social workers on this particular discharge planning task.

The independent variable of respondents tenure of employment and years of experience in discharge planning showed no association with their report of responsibility for advising patients of appeals or outcomes of appeals. The organization variable of auspice and size of hospital had no statistically significant relationship to the time spent on advising patients of the mechanism of appealing discharge decisions.

Another area of inquiry was to ask discharge planners if they found elderly patients asking for information about DRGs. The descriptive data showed no variation on this question. A comparison of nurses and social workers on this question finds them identical in their responses. Respondents stated that 63 percent of the time patients do not ask for information about DRGs, while one-third said 'yes, occasionally'.

Another question inquired whether discharge planners have to inform patients about DRGs and 61 percent of respondents answered affirmatively. This closely coincides with the previous question where 63 percent of patients do not inquire about DRGs. No significant difference appeared between nurses and social workers on this item.

The other area of generic inquiry on information about DRGs concerned the discharge planners' responsibility to inform consumers of DRGs. Social workers and nurses did not differ with any degree of statistical significance as to whose responsibility it is to inform consumers about DRGs. Indicating each agency which should take responsibility to inform the consumer, social workers and nurses responded similarly. it was no surprise that discharge planners felt that Medicare, more specifically the Health Care Finance Administration, (the organization responsible for implementing DRGs) should take the lead responsibility to inform consumers about DRGs. The discharge planners uniformly agree that both the New York City Department for the Aging and the media should be required to inform consumers before they are hospitalized and it then becomes the hospital's responsibility to provide such information.

Appeals of Discharge Decisions

Discharge planners were asked about the following three areas regarding patient appeals: 1) the frequency of appeals, 2) the most common types of situations which result in appeals and 3) outcomes of appeals.

In response to the first question, the response mean for nurses is 3.43 and quite similar for social workers, 3.41, which ranges between the 'occasionally' and 'frequently' in a range of 1 to 6 appeals per month. While almost one-quarter of the respondents 'do not know', the response of the 'others' tended to be in the middle range.

The variable of frequency of appeals, was correlated with auspice and bed size of the hospitals and no statistically significant differences were found between the three groups of hospitals and frequency of appeals.

One striking difference between nurses and social workers related to how they rank the most frequent situations which usually lead to appeals of discharge decisions. Nurses gave priority to the situation of 'patient/family feeling a longer stay in the hospital' (APPTYP2) is necessary as the 'most frequent' situation accounting for appeals. Social workers on the other hand rank the above, a longer hospital stay, as the least frequent situation. Social workers rank 'the nursing home of choice is not available' as the most frequent situation resulting in appeals. Nurses rank the latter as second most frequent.

The final aspect of appeals involved the discharge planners' awareness of the outcome of appeals. Almost 40 percent of respondents indicated they 'did not know' the outcome of appeals made by patients and/or their significant others. The findings indicate that both nurses and social workers tended to agree that outcomes of appeals generally favor the hospital, meaning the discharge decision was upheld. The differences between nurses and social workers responding to this question was not statistically significant utilizing the chi-square statistic.

Chapter 6

OBSTACLES TO DISCHARGE PLANNING

The obstacles to discharge planning attributable to the patient and/or their family and the reasons why the best discharge plans sometimes do not work out was elicited. Both nurses and social workers agree on the primary factor contributing to a 'good' discharge plan going awry, namely, that the family and/or patient are unrealistic in their expectations. Nurses ranked the patient's condition worsening as the second most frequent factor, while social workers identify inadequate home care availability as the second leading reason for discharge plans going awry. Lack of communication, primarily identified with physicians making decisions about discharge without consultation with other health care team members was the third factor identified by nurses and fourth most frequent factor identified by social workers. Nurses identified 'patient/family refusal to cooperate' as the fourth most frequent factor, while social workers ranked it eighth. Another area of difference between social workers and nurses relating to why discharge plans go awry is that there is limited nursing home bed availability. Nurses identify it as the fifth most frequent reason while social workers identify it as ninth.

This question of why discharge plans go awry was subsequently correlated with auspice and then with bed size of the hospital. Both variables showed no statistical significance in their relationship to why discharge plans go awry.

Another question asked respondents to rank in order of importance, the six factors which are most important for a 'successful' discharge plan. The theoretical score range is 1-6 with 1 being the most important factor. There was substantial agreement among the discharge planners who replied. They all agree on the first, second, and third factors namely, 'strong family support', 'the extent of patient's medical needs', and 'in-home service availability'. These factors support the frequency findings of high-risk screening criteria where 'family support criteria' are utilized for screening in over 70 percent of the hospitals. This has implications for the elderly, albeit a minority, who have no family supports and enter a hospital. The remaining three factors were mental status of patient, private financial resources and third party reimbursement.

Obstacles to discharge planning may occasionally be attributed to the patients themselves and their significant others. There are six commonly cited obstacles relating to patients and six stemming from their support network which were studied. Respondents scored responses on a scale of 1 to 4, where 1 equals never an obstacle and 4 equals frequently an obstacle.

Their assessment of patient-attributable obstacles to discharge planning are very similar. The rank order of patient obstacles to discharge planning are as follows: first, patient thinks Medicare covers more post hospital care than it does, second, patient not mentally able to cooperate, third, patient not physically able to cooperate, fourth, patient does not believe he/she will be discharged before ready, fifth, patient inflates level of support available post-discharge, and sixth, patient refuses to cooperate.

There is a modest difference between the frequency of ratings of discharge obstacles attributable to a patient's support network. Social workers most frequently reported the item family-related obstacles for discharge was that 'the support network was not realistic about discharge plans.' Nurses rank the item which states 'there is no available kith or kin' as the most frequent obstacle, while social workers rank it second. Nurses rank the item, 'the support network does not believe the patient will be discharged before he/she feels ready' as the second most frequent obstacle. Other items ranked as obstacles were 'not physically able to operate, not mentally able to cooperate, refusal to cooperate and does not believe patient will be discharged before he/she feels ready'.

Readmission Rates Since PPSs

Over 64 percent of respondents thought there was a higher rate of readmission of elderly persons since DRGs went into effect. While almost 25 percent report they did not know if the higher readmission rate among elderly persons was due to DRGs, only 10 percent report no increase in readmission of elderly patients.

Table 6-1 provides a comparison between nurses and social workers who reported an increase in the rate of readmission and the factors contributing to higher readmission among the elderly. Social workers viewed 'the current definition of skilled nursing as too restrictive for patients to receive adequate home care' as the leading factor. Nurses ranked this factor as third. Both nurses and social workers agree on the second factor namely, 'the inadequacy of in-home services available.'

Two variables reflected responses that are statistically significant between nurses and social workers. First is READMI5, 'the inadequate time for discharge planning.' Social workers were much more likely to report this as a factor contributing to readmissions of elderly patients since DRGs, than nurses. The mean for social workers is 3.15 in contrast to that of 4.88 for nurses ($t=2.77$; $p<0.009$).

'Overall impaired physical status of the patient,'(READMI6), was the second readmission variable with a significant difference between the two professional groups. This factor ranked first

TABLE 6-1
REASONS FOR RE-ADMISSIONS[t] BY RESPONDENT TYPE

Category of Re-admission Reasons	RESPONDENT TYPE							
	Nurse N=28			Social Worker N=198			T-VALUE	2-Tail Prob.
	Mean	S.D.	Rank	Mean	S.D.	Rank		
READMI 1	4.79	3.24	6	4.01	3.34	7	1.18	0.245
READMI 2	2.77	1.77	4	3.19	2.09	5	-1.10	0.280
READMI 3	2.38	1.84	2	2.61	1.73	2	-0.59	0.559
READMI 4	2.54	1.99	3	2.40	2.03	1	0.34	0.734
READMI 5	4.88	3.04	8	3.15	2.58	4	2.77	0.009*
READMI 6	1.92	1.67	1	2.76	2.20	3	-2.30	0.027*
READMI 7	3.19	1.96	5	3.63	2.57	6	-1.02	0.312
READMI 8	4.81	3.16	7	4.76	3.23	8	0.07	0.948

[t]Theoretical score range of 1-8 when 1 indicates highest frequency category for reasons of re-admission.

READMI 1 = Inadequate admission assessment
READMI 2 = Inadequate family support
READMI 3 = Inadequate in home services
READMI 4 = Inadequate definition of skilled care to receive in-home care
READMI 5 = Inadequate time for discharge planning
READMI 6 = Overall impaired physical status of patient
READMI 7 = Overall impaired mental status of patient
READMI 8 = Insufficient nursing home beds

*Statistically Significant

according to nurses with a mean of 1.92 in contrast to social workers with a mean of 2.76 (t=2.30; p<.027).

Nurses and Social Workers Performing Discharge Planning Tasks

This area of inquiry was adapted from a study comparing specific and overlapping functions and areas of collaborative activities between public health nurses and social workers (Robinson, 1967). Nine discharge planning functions had been identified and respondents asked to indicate whether the function, in order to obtain an optimal discharge plan, was best performed by: 1) collaboration, 2) either discipline, 3) nursing, or 4) social work.

In order to assess the magnitude of the association between the two nominal variables, namely, profession and discharge planning job functions, the nonparametric measure of correlation, the contingency coefficient (C) was employed. The purpose was to determine the probability associated with the occurrence of a correlation as large as the one observed in the sample under the null hypothesis that the variables are unrelated.

The chi-square statistic was employed to determine if the expected frequencies for each cell were significantly different than the observed frequencies. The larger the discrepancy between the expected values and the observed cell values, the larger is the degree of association between the two variables and thus the higher the value of C. The maximum value of C would fall just under 1.00 while no relationship would produce a contingency coefficient of zero. In determining the value of C, the chi-square statistic was computed and it also provided an adequate indication of the significance of C (Siegel, 1956).

The association of each of the nine discharge planning functions with the professions of nursing and social work were performed. The summary results of the primary domain attributed by each discipline to the nine discharge planning functions is presented in Table 6-2.

The majority (68%) of social workers perceived the discharge planning function of assessing a patient's support network as specifically or uniquely the domain of social work. Nurses predominantly perceived this function as either collaborative (50.0%) or discipline-appropriate among 36 percent of respondents. Slightly over 29 percent of social workers agree that this discharge planning function was collaborative while none felt it was unique to nursing. This situation offers a fertile ground for duplication of effort, competitive activity and feelings of intrusiveness by both groups of discharge planners. The remaining eight functions will be discussed which document five areas of agreement and three areas of disagreement.

TABLE 6-2
FUNCTIONS OF NURSES AND SOCIAL WORKERS AS PERCEIVED BY EACH GROUP

DISCHARGE PLANNING FUNCTION	NURSING	SOCIAL WORK
1. Assess Patient's Support Network	Collaborative	Social Work
2. Assess Patient's Home Environment	Collaborative/Either	Social Work
3. Assess Patient's Functional Status	Nursing	Collaborative
4. Initiate Referrals for Home Health	Nursing	Collaborative
5. Initiate Referrals for Home Care (non-health)	Social Work	Social Work
6. Identify Housing Options	Social Work	Social Work
7. Initiate Residential Placement	Social Work	Social Work
8. Discuss Financial Resources	Social Work	Social Work
9. Address Psychosocial Problems Related to Illness	Social Work	Social Work

The second discharge planning function looked at the responsibility for assessing a patient's home environment. Social workers perceived this discharge planning function as predominantly the domain of social work (65%) in contrast to nurses who divided their primary assignment between "collaborative" and "either," each with 29 percent of respondents. Twenty-five percent of the nurse professionals felt this function unique to nursing and 18 percent ascribed it to social work. Some social workers did agree with the collaborative area of practice as optimum (30%) and 7 percent felt either discipline could best perform the function. No social workers ascribed this area as unique to nursing. This documented another fertile area for role confusion between social workers and nurses performing discharge planning functions.

The third discharge planning function was assessing a patient's functional status and there was a relationship between the two variables. Given the nature of this variable, assessing functional status, it is no surprise that nurses feel it is overwhelmingly their domain (96%) with the remaining 4 percent indicating it could be either discipline. The majority of social workers feel it is a collaborative function (61%) with 32 percent perceiving it best handled by nursing. Either discipline was assigned by 4 percent of social work respondents and 3 percent of social workers felt it uniquely their own domain. Again, a very rich area for role controversy and turf issues to emerge between the two disciplines.

While not as strongly differentiated, the fourth discharge planning function showed the same trend as the previous one. The discharge planning function of referring to home health care is perceived by nursing to be primarily their domain among 67 percent of nurses. Social workers are more diverse in their perception of the domain in that this function was an area of collaborative practice (39%); a unique domain of social work (25%), and either discipline appropriate among 20 percent of social workers. Nurses in a smaller proportion do perceive this function as collaborative by 19 percent of discharge planners and equally between either discipline and uniquely social work among 7 percent of nurse respondents. The relation between professional discipline and the specific discharge planning function of initiating home health care referrals is C=0.37. Based on the chi-square ($x^2=36.5$; $p<0.001$), the contingency coefficient is statistically significant at the 0.001 level.

The next discharge planning function assessed the area of referring for non-health related home care. There was a relation between the variables of professional discipline and discharge planning function, C=0.32. It was statistically significant at the 0.001

level, (x^2=26.2; p<0.001). Social workers were much more in agreement than nurses on this function area. Social workers responses reflected 72 percent in agreement that this function is uniquely the domain of social work. This contrasts with nurses who perceive it to be a social work domain among 31 percent of respondents. Almost 27 percent of nursing respondents perceived it to be collaborative and equally as often to be optimum for either discipline to handle. Only 15 percent of nurses felt it to be uniquely the domain of nursing and only 2 percent of social workers attributed it to nursing. slightly over one quarter of the social work respondents felt this area could be carried out collaboratively or by either discipline. While social workers tend to be in agreement, nurses are much more varied as to their perception of whose discipline is most appropriate to have responsibility for this area of discharge planning.

The magnitude of association between professional discipline and area of discharge planning function is the lowest for the area of identifying housing options for patients. The contingency coefficient is 0.24 (x^2=30.9; p<0.004) and is statistically significant at the 0.01 level. Social workers and nurses are much more in agreement on the primary domain for this function being social work. Social workers perceive it 93 percent and nurses, 77 percent as social work's domain. No social workers perceive it as nursing's unique domain, and only 4 percent of nurses ascribe it to their own domain. Collaborative practice is perceived by nurses and social workers at 8 percent and 4 percent respectively.

Initiating residential placement applications on behalf of hospitalized patients is another domain of discharge planning examined. The relation between professional discipline and this discharge planning function is C=0.35 and it is statistically significant at the 0.001 level (x^2=30.9; $p<0.001$). Social workers perceive this as their unique domain (83%), while nurses perceive it as social work's domain 48 percent of the time. For 15 percent of the nurses and 12 percent of social workers it was perceived as a collaborative function. Nurses on the one hand, perceive it as either-discipline's domain among 30 percent of respondents. Both disciplines basically agree that it is not the domain of nursing to initiate residential placement.

Discussing financial resources related to discharge needs produces an association between this variable and professional discipline which is statistically significant (x^2=43.2; $p<0.001$). Over 92 percent of social workers perceive this function to be the domain of social work and just over half of the nurse respondents agree (52%). Nurses do perceive, with 30 percent frequency, that either discipline is appropriate in contrast to 3 percent of social work respondents who felt it to be either domain appropriate. With the large majority of social workers perceiving it as their primary domain, in contrast to nurses who only attribute it to social work half the time, this is another area of potential role confusion and potential duplication.

The last discharge planning function assessed which discipline is best equipped to address psychosocial problems related to illness. While 74 percent of social work respondents perceive this area unique to social work, nurses attribute it to social work by 37 percent of respondents which is about half being in agreement with social workers and half not. Nurses and social workers also favor collaborative practice in approximately one-quarter of responses. Nurses also perceive it to be either discipline's domain in 26 percent of responses while social workers do not agree and only attribute it to either discipline in 2.5 percent of responses. No social work respondents attribute this function of addressing psychosocial problems related to illness, to nurses.

The differences between nurses and social workers in their perception of the appropriate discipline, collaborative practice, or either discipline as optimum for discharge planning is statistically significantly different to warrant further attention.

Priorities for Professional Preparation

Discharge planners who indicated they had a professional discipline, were asked if they thought it prepared them adequately for discharge planning responsibilities. Less than half (46%) of all respondents replied that their professional school had prepared them adequately for discharge planning responsibilities. While social workers replied positively 46 percent of the time, nurses are slightly more favorable with 54 percent responding affirmatively about their professional training.

One-third of all respondents felt however that their professional school failed to prepare them adequately for discharge planning responsibilities. When looked at by professional discipline of nursing and social work, the findings were the same. One-third of the nurses and one-third of the social workers replied that their professional discipline did not adequately prepare them for discharge planning responsibilities.

Another area of inquiry focused on advice discharge planners would give to their professional school as to the types of skills needed for discharge planning. Responses were scored on a 5 point Likert scale, 1 being the lowest priority and 5 being the highest priority.

Priorities for eight skill areas identified by nurse and social worker respondents are reported in Table 6-3.

For both professional groups, all eight skill areas are given moderate to high priority. Six of the eight skill areas showed statistically significant differences between the two groups. On one hand, it may be argued that differences between nurses and social workers are to be expected; however, both nurses and social workers seem to be involved in what seems to be emerging as a new profession. Discharge planning personnel are beginning to refer to themselves as continuity of care professionals. If nurses were advising the curriculum, it appears that physical assessment and diagnostic skills would be the top priority among this respondent group. Social workers put this same skill area in a sixth position of priority. The scale means differ significantly on the physical assessment and diagnostic skill ($t=4.88$; $p<.001$).

Social workers rated counseling skills as their highest priority while nurses give it a significantly lower priority rating ($T=-3.45$; $p<0.002$). It should be pointed out that social workers and nurses did agree on the second priority area: mental assessment and diagnostic skill.

TABLE 6-3
PRIORITIES FOR PROFESSIONAL DISCIPLINE CURRICULA BY RESPONDENT TYPE

Skill Areas	RESPONDENT TYPE							T-VALUE	
	Nurse N=28			Social Worker N=198					
	Mean	S.D.	Rank	Mean	S.D.	Rank		T-VALUE	2-Tail Prob.
SKILL 1	4.64	0.68	1	3.89	1.16	6		4.99	0.000*
SKILL 2	4.46	0.79	2	4.56	0.72	2		-0.60	0.549
SKILL 3	3.89	0.83	7	4.39	0.85	4		-2.93	0.006*
SKILL 4	4.00	0.90	6	4.61	0.68	1		-3.45	0.002*
SKILL 5	4.22	0.85	4	4.54	0.65	3		-1.85	0.073
SKILL 6	3.04	1.07	8	3.62	1.03	8		-2.69	0.011*
SKILL 7	4.39	0.63	3	3.98	0.98	5		2.99	0.004*
SKILL 8	4.15	1.06	5	3.66	1.04	7		2.22	0.033*

SKILL 1 = Physical Assessment and Diagnostic
SKILL 2 = Mental Assessment and Diagnostic
SKILL 3 = Advocacy Skills
SKILL 4 = Counseling Skills
SKILL 5 = Collaborative Practice Skills
SKILL 6 = Financial Management
SKILL 7 = Health Care Policy
SKILL 8 = Medical Terminology

Scale Metrics: 1 = Low Priority; 2 = Moderately Low Priority; 3 = Moderate Priority; 4 = Moderately High Priority; and 5 = High Priority

*Statistical Significance

Advocacy skills, as perhaps might have been predicted, were given higher priority by social workers and result in a ranking of 4. Nurses rated it in seventh place. The differences between nurses and social workers on their priority for this skill was statistically significant (t=-2.93; p<0.006).

Collaborative practice skills were given similar priority by both professional respondents, however social workers gave slightly higher priority reflected by a mean of 4.54 which ranks third. The mean score on collaborative practice skills among nurses is 4.22, resulting in a rank of 4.

Nurses gave the curriculum area of 'health care policy' quite a high priority reflected by a mean of 4.39. Health care policy resulted in a rank of 3 among the eight identified curriculum areas among nurses. Social workers gave this area a lower priority than nurses. The difference between social workers and nurses on this area of priority for their professional school curriculum was statistically significant (t=-2.99; p<0.004).

The curriculum area of medical terminology was given higher priority by nurses than by social workers. This is not surprising since the discipline of nursing is based in part on the science of medicine. It is interesting to note that the initial training inaugurated for social workers (friendly visitors) in hospitals in the early 1920s also included this curriculum component.

128 Prospective Payments and Discharge Planning

Inclusion of medical terminology in medical social work training continued until the late 1940s when more generic social work education prevailed (Cannon, 1913; Rehr,1983). The difference in mean scores between nurses and social workers was statistically significant ($t=2.22, p<0.33$).

The lowest priority area for both disciplines was that of financial management. Both groups obviously recognize its importance since the mean scores fell in the 'moderate priority range. The difference between the mean scores was statistically significant ($t=2.69; p<0.011$).

A respondent's employment tenure at the hospital and years of discharge planning experience had no impact on discharge planner priority areas for school curricula. The auspice and the hospital size which respondents represented had no significance either.

Personnel Changes Due to PPS

Timely discharges were a more critical concern with the Prospective Payment System because each unnecessary day in the hospital diminished the profit or increased the loss per patient. While many hospitals were containing costs by reducing staff, it was anticipated that due to the increased emphasis on discharge planning, there would be an increase in discharge planning personnel. One limitation of this question is that there are no comparative data for other unit/divisions at the hospital nor any comparative staff size data prior to DRG implementation.

There was a statistically significant difference in how nurses and social workers responded to the question of whether there had been any changes in discharge planning staff at their hospital attributable to DRGs ($t=2.86$; $p<0.007$). While 64 percent of the nurses indicated a staff increase, only 32 percent of social workers reported staff increases due to DRGs. Discharge planners who were nurses reported no staff decrease while social workers reported staff decreased by 16 percent due to DRGs.

Chapter 7

CONCLUSIONS

This study met its broad research objectives of determining a number of effects caused by the new prospective payment reimbursement policy on discharge planners with the elderly in New York City acute care hospitals. The limitations of this type of study are that standardized questionnaires at a point in time cannot capture the total milieu of hospital discharge planners. Survey research can only collect self-reports of recalled past actions or prospective action (Babbie, 1986).

Sampling the universe of acute care hospital discharge planners in New York City raises several questions about the non-respondents. What was the professional discipline of non-respondent discharge planners? If all were nurses, it may substantiate the view of key informants that discharge planners are more evenly divided between nurses and social workers than this study revealed. The site visit to one hospital and the in-depth interviews with the site-hospital staff helps to overcome some of the limitations of survey research by providing a more dynamic sense of the impact of the Prospective Payment System on the discharge planning function.

This study examined the task responsibilities of personnel providing discharge planning services to the elderly and the impact of DRGs on their work. Differences between nurses and social workers performing parallel discharge planning functions and the areas of potential duplication were identified. The extent to which obstacles to discharge planning were exacerbated by DRGs was also documented. Changes in the organization of discharge planning activities and staffing patterns, in addition to specific service need changes attributable to DRGs were identified. The role of discharge planners to inform patients of their right to appeal discharge plans was presented and their perceptions of the reasons for appeal, the extent of appeal, and the perception of appeal outcomes were examined.

Among the key independent variables, professional discipline, specifically nursing and social work, and the Prospective Payment System, proved to be the most significant. The data support an overall constellation of increased job responsibilities among discharge planners resulting from DRGs. Nurses reported greater change in the time spent on various discharge planning tasks. All respondents felt there was less time for supervision and teaching of student professionals and more time was spent on screening and interviewing patients for post-hospital discharge planning needs. Social workers reported having less time to do counseling tasks with patients and their families while nurses reported a counseling increase.

According to the data, discharge planners felt negatively about DRGs and their impact on the elderly. There was one area of exception. Some nurses did feel DRGs had enhanced their role status among hospital personnel.

Nearly 50 percent of the discharge planners felt their professional education prepared them inadequately for discharge planning responsibilities and have recommendations for their professional schools.

The demographic reality of an aging population is here. This fastest growing segment of the population presents a challenge to all health professions. It is imperative that professional schools prepare the next generation of social workers and nurses to meet the discharge planning requirements of the elderly as they adapt to illness and the concomitant functional losses. While discharge planning for a patient's post-hospital care is only one aspect of services in a hospital setting, it is a critical one.

The site visit and key informant data sources portrayed cause for alarm in the future recruitment of social workers for work in hospitals. The syndrome of discharging patients 'quicker and sicker' and the overwhelming perception that elderly patients are readmitted more frequently since DRG implementation, lends support to this concern. In addition, fiscal constraints have changed the nature of discharge planning tasks in ways which threaten the quality of social work services in health care.

The disparity in the assignment of role domains between nurses and social workers needs attention. The ability to define the functions of discharge planning which are unique to nursing, unique to social work, either-discipline appropriate, or best performed collaboratively, needs clarification. While social workers seem to be less inclined than nurses to collaborative practice, both disciplines do rate 'collaborative practice skills' as a priority recommendation for professional training. Priorities for professional school curricula differed significantly in this study between nurses and social workers. Nurses gave top priority to physical assessment and diagnostic skills while social workers rated counseling skills foremost. The skill area of advocacy earned a rank of four among social workers and a rank of seven among nurses. The area of health care policy was ranked third by nurses and fifth by social workers.

Areas for Further Study

Five areas for further inquiry have been identified as a result of this study. The first is a need for a factual survey of how discharge planning is organized in acute care hospitals. What are the differences in organizational structure for those units under the direction of nurses and those under the direction of social workers? How are roles delineated and what is the interface of social work and nursing in role functions in each structure? Such an inquiry should also obtain from hospital administration its understanding of role delineations for discharge planning.

A qualitative study of readmissions among elderly persons is needed to document the perceptions among discharge planners that the rate of readmissions is much higher since DRGs. Deciphering what are most likely a very complex set of reasons for readmissions would put to rest, or support, the allegation that DRGs are responsible for 'irresponsible' discharging of older adults who are simply not well enough to return to the community.

Key informants constantly reiterated that it is more and more difficult to recruit social workers to work in hospitals. Research is needed to understand why 'burnout' is occurring. Site visit respondents felt that social work in hospitals has become more like a job of constant crisis intervention and that the variety of social service activities, historically part of medical social work, have been overwhelmed by discharge planning responsibilities. This warrants attention.

Almost seventy percent of the discharge planners do not supervise professional students. Given the impression that it is becoming more difficult to attract social workers to hospital settings and particularly discharge planning, this area needs to be studied in conjunction with the above concern and in partnership with professional schools. The final area of research is one of assessing whether discharge planning is becoming or should become a professional specialization. The trend seems to be toward the development of a continuity of care professional discipline, as the objectives of the American Association of Continuity of Care reflect. It seems appropriate for the disciplines of nursing and social work to proactively assess this trend and qualitatively review their own curricula to determine if, in addition, there is a need for a discharge planning specialization within their disciplines.

Educational and Policy Development

Several areas of research identified in the above sections have educational implications for the professional training of social workers and nurses. Documentation is provided by the survey data that points toward duplication of effort, competitive activity and feelings of intrusiveness between social workers and nurses. The lack of consensus between social workers and nurses as to whose domain several key discharge planning functions belong, may lead to unsatisfactory professional relationships and poor work on behalf of patients and their families. A productive relationship, as observed in the site visit, depends on the extent of understanding each group has of its own functions, recognition by both disciplines of their common interest and skills, and an appreciation of the unique contributions each has to offer (Robinson, 1967).

Professional schools need to teach students how to clearly delineate roles, and how to collaborate with other professional disciplines. Such learning begins with a firm foundation in the profession's own theory and practice and moves to an understanding of other professions. A course or unit on the sociology of professions would provide a base from which students could begin to understand the similarities and differences of professions.

As a related educational recommendation, greater emphasis must be placed on each profession's code of ethics. Concern for social workers employed in host settings, such as hospitals is not new. Responsibility and allegiance to the client is in conflict with the host agency at times. No clearer case is required to document this point than the data findings of this research. Discharge planners do not see as their role the responsibility for advising patients of the appeals mechanism. When this question was probed during the site visit, social workers reported that it was their job to work with patients and families to avoid appeals and that it was the responsibility of the patient advocate to intervene if the patient appealed. The mandate is clear for educators.

Interdisciplinary practice is, of

course, essential in health care settings and there is an increased educational need for skills in communication with other disciplines and work in collaborative practice. Since physicians were cited as the worst offenders, medical school educators as well as hospital administrators should heed the problem and work toward enhancing communication among the hospital's multiple disciplines for the benefit of the patient as well as for themselves.

The major policy recommendations emerging from this research relate to the continuum of care for older adults. In a move to contain costs at the most expensive level (the hospital), the Prospective Payment System was introduced. This system has shortened the average hospital 'length of stay' among older adults, yet the system gives no recognition to the need to enhance community based services while implicitly increasing the burden such services need to bear. Instead, further fiscal austerity has been applied to home health care benefits available under Medicare with a reduction in covered services. A major reemphasis on community based services is required, with a funding mechanism which recognizes the chronic nature of services most often required by the elderly, rather than the acute care medical model fostered by Medicare in 1965.

The data support the increased need for case management services among the elderly discharged to community care. The finding that Visiting Nurse Services are the most frequent referral source for case management is cause for some alarm. Visiting Nurse Services have a limited number of social workers on their staffs, and in 1986-87 terminated the employment of all social workers in Manhattan and the Bronx when they faced fiscal difficulties: and, by the nature of their reliance on Medicare reimbursement, they have very restrictive guidelines for how long they may serve a patient under this reimbursement source. What are the options for provision of case management service? Other than social security benefits, the Older Americans Act does not have adequate funding support to undertake case management services, although they do provide this service in many of their funded programs. Given the demographic bulge and the increased number of frail, old-old persons, the coverage of case management is imperative under both Medicare and Medicaid programs.

Specific to the Prospective Payment System, is the need for recognition of individual differences in the factors which combine to establish a fixed rate of reimbursement for each Diagnosis Related Grouping. This could be accommodated if modifications to the severity-of-illness index were made and the requirement established that discharge planners assess the unique factors which coalesce to potentially make a discharge plan unsafe for patients.

Discharge planners cannot be the pawns for the implementation of discharge plans which they professionally judge to be ill advised or unsafe. The implications of how health care professionals are responding to legislative mandates such as the Prospective Payment System which tend to place too much emphasis on cost containment at the expense of quality of care and concern for the individual patient should be given further attention.

EPILOGUE

Discharge planning continues to be an important focus of attention in the 1990s following the implementation of the Prospective Payment System for reimbursing hospital costs of Medicare-eligible persons in the mid-1980s. This dramatic new method of reimbursement based on DRGs is not only being implemented in the United States but in various configurations throughout Europe, Scandinavia and Australia (Bardsley et al, 1987).

The Health Care Financing Administration proposed new rules in 1988 regarding standards for discharge planning for Medicare beneficiaries (Federal Registry, 1988). These standards included identification, evaluation, formal written discharge plan, continuity of information transfer, and reassessment to be performed by an interdisciplinary team. Discharge planning is now seen as an entitlement for all Medicare-eligible hospitalized patients and makes the documentation of discharge plans a requirement for Medicare reimbursement. Five variables are used to set the payment rate for a given patient in a given hospital: the location of the hospital (urban versus rural); hospital wages in the area; the patient's diagnosis-related group; the size of the hospital's teaching program; and the share of low-income patients served by the hospital. Additional payments are made if the patient is an outlier, that is, has an exceptionally long stay or high costs. Some argue that the system still does not adequately account for the patient's severity of illness (Russell, 1989).

A number of concerns continue to be raised about the impact of a Prospective Payment System on the health of older adults. There is now some data to look at mortality rates, average length of stay and readmission rates to hospitals.

Mortality rates have not shown any clear trend since the inauguration of PPS. There have been fluctuations since 1983 starting with a slight decline, a rise in between 1984 and 1985, and a return in 1986 to the level of 1984 (National Center for Health Statistics, 1987). This bears monitoring.

The average length of stay in hospitals has gradually declined over the past twenty years. In 1968, the average length of stay for a Medicare-eligible person age 65 and over was 13.8 days, in 1983 it had dropped to 9.7 days; and in 1988 it was 8.8 days (Bureau of Census, 1972-88).

The inspector general of the Department of Health and Human Services studied a Medicare sample of more than 7,000 hospital admissions to check for premature discharges in the first year of PPS implementation and found that less than 1% were discharged prematurely (Office of Inspector General,1988). Professional Review Organizations are charged with reviewing a sample of readmissions up to 31 days of discharge; however not much of their data has yet been released. Readmission statistics do not reveal any clear signs of deterioration in quality (Russell, 1989).

One study found that the number of older adults admitted to hospitals via the emergency room has risen significantly since the implementation of DRGs which warrants further study (Sloan et al 1988). Another study of 648 internists of the American Society of Internal Medicine (ASIM, 1988) found that 55% of the respondents had experienced pressure to delay admitting patients to the hospital until the patient was sick enough to meet the requirements of the Peer Review Organization (PRO). Half of the internists acknowledged that a positive effect of DRGs was in reducing unnecessary hospitalization as well as tests and procedures.

Assessing the patients perceptions of their care in hospitals under PPS reveals conflicting opinions. Fischer and Eustis (1988) asked patients and families their impression of medical care before and after the implementation of DRGs. They found that respondents were much more concerned with quality of care and cited examples of inadequate provision of care. Monk and Stuen (1988) in a study that interviewed patients thirty days post discharge from three New York City hospitals found them to be generally satisfied with services they received in the hospital.

Being prematurely discharged in a more frail, sick state of health without adequate community supports remains a major concern for older adults, health care workers and policymakers. The study of internists and other interviews with patients and/or their families have provided case material documenting incidents of the 'discharge quicker and sicker' syndrome and its potential deleterious consequences for older adults (ASIM, 1988; Coulton, 1988; Fischer and Eustis, 1988; and Mizrahi, 1988).

Issues of dual loyalty are intensified for hospital discharge planners who work in this era of cost-containment. Nurses and social workers have professional codes of ethics which requires them to keep the patient's interests primary while their hospital administrators are pressuring for conservation of hospital resources. Social workers have practiced in diverse host settings since the profession's origins; settings in which social workers practice is defined and dominated by people who are not social workers (Dane and Simon, 1991). Davidson (1978) cautioned social workers involved in hospital discharge planning to retain their primary role of service to the individual client. "In hospitals...timely assessment and discharge planning appear to be the central tasks for social workers. If the physician or hospital administrator wants to discharge the patient before community resources are in place, ethical problems arise for the social worker who is asked to implement this decision" (Dane and Simon, 1991, p.209). This same conflict would exist for nurses who work as discharge planners also.

The need to increase communication among the interdisciplinary team members involved in patient care was documented by this study and others subsequently (Bull, 1988; Wertheimer and Kleinman, 1990). This study also documented areas of role confusion and turf concerns between nurses and social workers involved in discharge planning. The potential for conflict is present among the myriad of disciplines comprising the interdisciplinary health care team and needs to be addressed and channelled to allow for maximizing the patient's and the community's resources to insure a safe, responsible discharge from the hospital. Many hospitals are now adding a variety of outpatient and community-based services to their organizations such as home care, nursing home care, social work consultation for physicians, case management services, and development of health education and promotion programs (Blumenfield and Rosenberg, 1988). This helps to insure that the patient will have the resources needed upon discharge without dependency on other service providers and offers other reimbursement streams for the hospital's economic survival.

The American Association for Continuity of Care has moved ahead with a program to train and certify discharge planners. This seems to be a direct response to the feelings expressed by this study and others that professionals engaged in discharge planning did not feel adequately prepared for their work by their professional school's curriculum. Social work and nursing educators need to take heed to this phenomenon or else a new professional discipline will evolve to meet this growing demand for discharge planning services.

BIBLIOGRAPHY

Abramson, M. 1981. Ethical Dilemmas for Social Workers in Discharge Planning, **Social Work and Health Care**, 6, pp. 33-41.

American Association of Continuity of Care. 1984. **Turf Problems**, Task Force Report. Washington, DC: American Association of Continuity of Care.

American Nurses Association. 1979. **A Case for Baccalaureate Preparation in Nursing**. New York: American Nurses Association.

American Nurses Association. 1964. **Educational Preparation for Nurse Practitioners and Assistants of Nurses: A Position Paper**. New York: American Nurses Association.

American Society of Internal Medicine. (1985). **The Impact of DRG's on Patient Care**. Washington, DC.

Argyris, C. 1964. **Integrating the Individual and the Organization**. New York: Wiley.

Austin, C.D. 1983. Case Management in Long Term Care: Options and Opportunities, **Health and Social Work**, 8(1), pp. 16-30.

Babbie, E.R. 1975. **The Practice of Social Research**. Belmont, CA: Wadsworth Publishing, Inc.

Bailis, S.S. 1985. A Case for Generic Social Work in Health Settings, **Social Work**, 30(3), pp. 209-213.

Bardsley, M., Coles, J., Jenkins, L. 1987. **DRGS and Health Care**. London: Kings Fund Publishing Office.

Barker, R.L. and Briggs, T.L. 1968. **Differential Use of Social Work Manpower**. New York: National Association of Workers.

Barrow, R.N. 1978. The Present Role of the Nurse in the Delivery of Health Care. In **The Changing Role of Health Care Personnel Worldwide in View of the Increase of Basic Health Services.** R.W. McNeur, Ed. Philadelphia, PA: Society for Health and Human Values.

Bartlett, H.M. 1975. Ida M. Cannon: Pioneer in Medical Social Work. **Social Service Review**, 49(2), p. 12.

Bartlett, H.M. 1978. **Social Work Practice in the Health Field.** New York: National Association of Social Workers.

Batey, M.V. and Lewis, F.M. 1982. Clarifying Autonomy and Accountability in Nursing Service. **Journal of Nursing Administration**, 12(9), p. 15.

Beale, P. and Gulley, M. 1981. Discharge Planning Process: An Interdisciplinary Approach. **Military Medicine**, 146 (10), pp. 713-716.

Berkman, B.G. 1970. **Social Service Casefinding with Hospitalized Elderly.** Doctoral Dissertation, Columbia University.

Berkman, B.G. 1978. Knowledge Base and Program Needs for Effective Social Work Practice in Health Care: A Review of the Literature, Society for Hospital Social Work Directors. Chicago, IL: American Hospital Association.

Berkman, B.G. and Rehr, H. 1973. Early Social Service Case Finding for Hospitalized Patients: An Experiment, **Social Service Review**, 47, pp. 256-265.

Black, B. 1971. Social Work in Health and Mental Health Services. **Social Casework**, 52 pp. 211-219.

Black, R.B. 1984. Looking Ahead: Social Work as a Core Health Profession, **Health and Social Work**, 9(2), pp. 85-95.

Black R.B., Dornan, D.H. and Allegrante, J.P. 1986. Challenges in Developing Health Promotion Services for the Chronically Ill. **Social Work**, 31 (4), pp. 287-293.

Blake, R. 1980. Hospital Social Work: What is Needed are Results, **Social Work**, 25(5), pp. 411-412.

Blazyk, S. and Canavan, M.M. 1985. Therapeutic Aspects of Discharge Planning, **Social Work**, 30(6), pp. 489-496.

Blumenfield, S. and Rosenberg, G. 1988. Towards a Network of Social Health Services: Redefining Discharge Planning and Expanding the Social Work Domain. Social Work in Health Care, 13, 31-48.

Bogdan, R. and Taylor, S. 1975. **Introduction to Qualitative Research Methods.** New York: John Wiley and Sons.

Boone, C.R., Coulton, C., and Keller, S. 1971. The Impact of Early and Comprehensive Social Work Services on Length of Stay, **Social Work in Health Care**, 7, pp. 1-9.

Borland, J.J. and Strauss, M. 1982. Social Work Education for Health Care: A Blueprint for Action, **Social Work**, 7(3), pp. 224-229.

Bull, M.J. 1988. Influence of Diagnosis-Related Groups on Discharge Planning, Professional Practie, and Patient Care. Journal of Professional Nursing, 4, 412-421.

Burack-Weiss, A. 1986. Helping Elders Use Help: A clinical Perspective on Case Management. Paper presented Brookdale Institute Spring Seminar Series, Columbia University, April 9, 1986.

Bureau of Census. 1972-1988. **Statistical Abstract of the United States.** Washington, D.C.

Burling, T., Lentz, E.M., and Wilson, R.N. 1956. **The Give and Take in Hospitals: A Study of Human Organizations in Hospitals.** New York: G.P. Putnam's Sons.

Burnham, J.C. 1982. American Medicine's Golden Age: What Happened to It? **Science,** 215(March 19), pp. 1474-1479.

Bracht, N.F. 1974. Health Care: The Largest Human Service System, **Social Work,** 19(5), pp. 532-543.

Bracht, N.F. ed. 1978. **Social Work in Health Care: A Guide to Professional Practice.** New York: Haworth Press.

Brandon, R.M. 1986. Organizing for Health Care Reform, **Social Policy,** 17(2) pp. 57-58.

Brochstein, J., Adams, G., Tristan, M., and Chaney, C. 1979. Social Work and Primary Care: An Integrative Approach, **Social Work in Health Care,** 5(1).

Brody, E.M. 1981. The Dependent Elderly and Women's Changing Chaning Roles, **Mt. Sinai Journal of Medicine,** 48(6), pp. 511-519.

Brody, H. 1973. The Systems View of Man: Implications for Medicine, Science and Ethics, **Perspectives in Biology and Medicine**, Fall, pp. 71-92.

Brody, S. 1980. Health Care for the Aged, **Hospitals**, 54(10), pp. 63-66.

Brody, S. and Persily, N. 1984. **Hospitals and the Aged.** Rockville, MD: Aspen.

Cannon, I.M. 1913. **Social Work in Hospitals.** New York: Russell Sage Foundation.

Capitman, J.A., Haskins, B. and Bernstein, J. 1986. Case Management Approaches in Coordinated Community Oriented Long-Term Care Demonstrations, **The Gerontologist,** 26(4), pp. 398-404.

Caputi, M.A. 1982. A 'Quality of Life' Model for Social Work Practice in Health Care, **Health and Social Work,** 7(2), pp. 103-110.

Caputi, M.A. and Heiss, W.A. 1984. The DRG Revolution, **Health and Social Work,** 9(1), pp. 5-12.

Carlton, T.O. 1984. **Clinical Social Work in Health Setting.** New York: Springer Publishing Co.

Carr-Saunders, A.M. 1955. Metropolitan Conditions and Traditional Professional Relations. In **The Metroplis in Modern Life R.M. Fisher**, Ed., New York: Doubleday, pp. 279-287.

Chelimsky, E. 1985. Evaluating the Effects of Medicare Prospective Payment on Post-Hospital Care, Statement before Special Senate Committee on Aging. Washington, DC: United States GAO.

Chelimsky, E. 1985. Information Requirements for Evaluating the Impact of Medicare Prospective Payment on Post-Hospital Long Term Care Services: Preliminary Report (GAO/PEMD-85-8). Letter to Special Committee on Aging, U.S. Senate.

Chisholm, M.M. 1983. Promises and Pitfalls of Discharge Planning, **Nursing Management**, 14(11), pp. 26-29.

Christ, W. 1984. Factors Delaying Discharge of Psychiatric Patients, **Health and Social Work**, 9(3), pp. 178-187.

Clark, P.G. 1984. The Social Allocation of Health Care Resource: Ethical Dilemmas in Age-Group competition, **The Gerontologist**, 25, pp. 119-125.

Clausen, C. 1984. Staff RN: A Discharge Planner for Every Patient, **Nursing Management**, 15(11), pp. 58-61.

Cochrane, E. 1981. Discharge Planning: The Central Role of Social Work, **NASW News**, 26 February, p.14.

Cohen, J. 1965. Statistical Issues in Psychosocial Research, in **Handbook of Clinical Psychological Research**, B.B. Wolman, Ed., New York: McGraw-Hill.

Cohen, J. 1977. **Statistical Power Analysis for the Behavioral Sciences**, Revised Edition. New York: Academic Press.

Collins, M. 1977. **Communication in Health Care**. Saint Louis: The C.V. Mosby Co.

Committee on Function of Nursing. 1948. **A Program for the Nursing Profession**. New York: The MacMillan Co.

Congressional Budget Office. February, 1984. **Reducing the Deficit: Spending and Revenue Options,** Part 3. Washington, D.C.: Congressional Budget Office.

Congressional Record 1967. Expansion and development of Social Work Manpower Training, 19th Congress, 1st Session, 113, No. 33, p. 52495 (Bill No. 1150).

Continuity of Care Management: New Concepts in Hospital Admissions/Discharge Planning. (1984). Albany: New York State Health Planning Commission, Staff Paper.

Coughlin B.J. 1970. Reconceptualizing the Theorectical Base of Social Work Practice. In **Innovations in Teaching Social Work Pracatice,** L. Ripple, Ed. New York: Council on Social Work Education.

Coulton, C.J. 1979. **Social Work Quality Assurance Programs: A Comparative Analysis.** Washington, DC: National Association of Social Workers.

Coulton, C.J. 1981. Person-environment Fit as a Focus in Health Care, **Social Work,** 26(1), pp. 26-35.

Coulton, C.J. 1984. Confronting Prospective Payment: Requirements for an Information System. **Health and Social Work,** 9(1), pp. 13-24.

Coulton, C.J., Dunkle, R.E., Goode, R.A., and MacKintosh, J. 1982. Discharge Planning and Decision Making, **Health and Social Work,** 7(3), pp. 253-261.

Craig, S. 1985. On American Association of Continuity of Care, **ACCESS**, 5(5), pp. 2.

Crumpton, P.A. 1986. The Issue of Turf, **The Next Step: The Glasrock Home Health Care Newsletter for Discharge Planning,** 3(1), p. 4

Curran, C. and Metcalf, C. 1983. Combining Resource, **Nursing Management,** 14(1), pp. 33-39.

Curtin, L.L. 1986. Nursing in the Year 2000: Learning from the Future (Editorial Opinion) **Nursing Management,** 17(6), pp. 7-8.

Dana, B. 1983. The Collaborative Practice. In **Social Work Issues in Health Care,** H. Rehr and R. Miller, Ed. Englewood Cliffs, N.J.: Prentice-Hall, Inc.

Dane, B.O. Simmon, B.L. 1991. Resident Guests: Social Workers in Hospital Settings. **Social Work,** 36(3), pp 208-213.

Davidson, K.W. 1978. Evolving Social Work Roles in Health Care: The Case of Discharge Planning. **Social Work in Health Care,** 4, 43-53.

Davis, C.K. 1983. The Federal Role in Changing Health Care Financing, **Nursing Economics,** 1, pp. 98-104.

Davis K. and Schoen, C. 1978. **Health and War on Poverty: A Ten Year Appraisal.** Washington, DC: The Brookings Institution.

Demos, J. 1970. **A Little Commonwealth.** New York: Oxford University Press.

Department of Health, Education and Welfare. 1963. Toward Quality in Nursing: Needs and Goals, Report of the Surgeon General's Consultant Group on Nursing. Washington, DC: U.S. Government Printing Office.

DiNitto, D.M. and Dye, T.R. 1983. **Social Welfare: Politics and Public Policy.** Englewood Cliffs, N.J.: Prentice-Hall.

Donabedian, A. 1982. Models for Organizing the Delivery of Personal Health Services and Criteria for Evaluating Them, **Milbank Memorial Fund Quarterly,** Vol. L(4), P. 107.

Ell, K. and Morrison, D. 1981. Primary Care, **Health and Social Work,** Supplement on Specialization and Special Interests, 6(4).

Epstein, I. 1970. Professionalization, Professionalism and Social Worker Radicalism, **Journal of Health and Human Behavior,** 11(1), pp. 67-78.

Etzioni, A. (Ed.) 1969. **The Semi-Professions and Their Organization.** New York: The Free Press.

Evashwick, C.J., Rundell, T., and Goldiamond, B. 1985. Hospital Services for Older Adults, **The Gerontologist,** 25(6), pp. 631-637.

Feather, J. 1985. Megacorporate Health Care: Is It Good for the Elderly? The Case of Discharge Planning, Paper presented at the New York State Gerontological Educators Annual Meeting, October 9-11.

Federal Council on Aging 1981. Sources of Payment for Hospital Care for Population 65+, 1980. **The Need for Long Term Care: Information and Issues.** Washington, DC: U.S. Department of Health and Human Services.Federal Registry. 1988, June. **Health Care Finance Administration Proposed Regulations for Discharge Planning.** pp. 22506-22509.

Feldman, J. and Goldhaber, F. 1984. Living With DRGs, **Journal of Nursing Administration**, 14, pp. 19-22.

Fischer, L. R. , and Eustis, N.N. 1988. DRGs and Family Care for the Elderly: A Case Study. **The Gerontologist**, 28, 383-389.

Fox, R.C. 1977. The Medicalization and Demedicalization of American Society, **Daedalus**, 106, p. 21.

Flexner, A. 1915. **Is Social Work a Profession?** New York: The New York School of Philanthropy.

Foster, Z. and Brown, D.L. 1978. The Social Work Role in Hospital Discharge Planning: An Administrative Case History, **Social Work in Health Care**, 4, pp.55-63.

Frangos, A. and Chase, D. 1976. Potential Partners: Attitudes of Family Practice Residents Toward Collaboration with Social Workers in Their Future Practice, **Social Work in Health Care**, 2(67).

French, L.M. 1940. **Psychiatric Social Work.** New York: Commonwealth Fund.

Friedson, E. 1959. Specialties Without Roots: The Utilization of New Services, **Human Organization**, 18, pp. 112-116.

Friedson, E, 1970. **Profession of Medicine: A Study of the Sociology of Applied Knowledge.** New York: Dodd, Mead and Company.

Garner, J.D. and Mercer, S.O. 1982. Meeting the Needs of the Elderly: Home Health Care or Institutionalization? **Health and Social Work**, 7(3), pp. 183-191.

Gartner, A. 1976. **The Preparation of Human Service Professionals.** New York: Human Sciences Press.

Gaynor, Jr. J.M., Kast, D. A., and Mills, E.M. 1984. DRG's: Regulatory and Budgetary Adjustments. **Nursing and Health Care**, 5, pp. 275-278.

Germain, C.B. 1984. **Social Work Practice In Health Care: An Ecological Perspective.** New York: The Free Press.

Gibson, R.M. and Waldo, D.R. 1981. National Health Expenditures, 1980, **Health Care Financing Review.** HCFA Publication No. 03123. Health Care Financing Administration, Office of Research, Demonstration and Statistics. Washington, DC: U.S. Government Printing Office.

Ginzberg, E. 1981. Large-Scale Growth in Health Dollars Attracts Attention of For-Profit Sector, **Hospitals**, July 16, 55(14), pp. 90-93

Ginzberg, E. 1982. Competition in Health Care: A Second Opinion, **Hospitals**, March 16, 56(6), p. 81.

Goldberg, E.M. and Neil, J.E. 1972. **Social Work in General Practice.** London: George Allen and Univin.

Goldstein, D. 1954. **Readings in the Theory and Practice of Medical Social Work.** Chicago: University of Chicago Press.

Goode, W.J. 1957. Community Within a Community: The Professions, **American Socialogical Review,** 22(2), pp. 194-200.

Gordon, B. and Rehr, H.1969. Selectivity Biases in Delivery of Hospital Social Services, **Social Service Review,** 43 (1), pp.35-41.

Gordon, E. 1954. **Medical Social Work Looks at Nursing Education.** A report prepared under the supices of a subcommittee of the Education Committee of the American Association of Medical Social Workers.

Grimaldi, P.L. 1983. New Medicare DRG Payment Calculations Issued, **Nursing Management,** 14(1), pp. 19-23.

Grimaldi, P.L. 1983. Public Law 97-248: The Implications of Prospective Payment Schedules, **Nursing Management,** 14(2), pp.25-27.

Grimaldi, P.L. 1986. New Legislation Tightens PPS, **Nursing Management,** 17(6), pp.20-22.

Grossman, L., Harrell, W., and Melamed, M. 1979. Changing Hospital Practice and Social Work Staffing, **Social Work,** 5, pp.411-415.

Gurin, A. and Williams, D. 1973. Social Work Education, In **Education for the Professions of Medicine, Law, Technology and Social Work,** Everett C. Hughes. New York: McGraw-Hill.

Hallowitz, E. 1972. Innovations in Hospital Social Work, **Social Work**, 17, pp.89-97.
Hamilton, J.M. 1984. Nursing and DRGs: Proactive Responses to Prospective Reimbursement, **Nursing and Health Care**, 5(3), pp.155-159.
Hanson, P. C. 1985. **Management Systems for the Discharge Planning Professional.** Eagan, MN: Healthcare Management Services.
Hardy, M.E. 1978. **Role Theory: Perspectives for Health Professionals.** New York: Appleton-Century-Crofts.
Harlow, K.S. and Wilson, L.B. 1985. Community Services Hit Heavy by DRGs, **Coordinator**, 4(9), pp.29-31.
Harrington, C. 1985. Crisis in Long TermCare: Part 1, The Problems, **Nursing Economics**, 3(1), pp.15-20.
Harrington, C. 1985. Crisis in Long Term Care: Part 2, Policy Options, **Nursing Economics**, 3(2), pp.109-115.
Health Care Finance Administration. 1983. **The Medicare and Medicaid Data Book 1983.** Baltimore, Md: Health Care Finance Administration.
Health Care Finance Administration. 1985. Report on PPS Monitoring Activities, Memorandum, January 20, 1985.
Health Facilities in Southern New York. 1985. He alth Care Information Series. New York: United Hospital Fund.
Herzog, A.R. and Dielman, L. 1985. Age Differences in Response Accuracy for Factual Survey Questions, **Journal of Gerontology**, 40(3), pp.350-357.
Holt, R.H. 1982. Occupational Stress. In **Handbook of Stress**, L. Goldberger and Breznitz, Eds. New York: Free Press.

Holzener, W.L. and Anderson, M. 1982. Articulation in Baccalaureate Nursing Education. In **Nursing Education**, M.S. Henderson, Ed. London: Churchill Foundation.

Hookey, P. 1976. Social Education for the Field of Health, **Social Work in Health Care**, 1(3), pp.337-345.

Horejsi, G.A. 1983. Group Discharge Planning, **Health and Social Work**, 8(3), p.245.

Houston, L.S. and Cadenhead, G. 1986. DRGs and BSNs: The Case for the Baccalaureate Nurse, **Nursing Management**, 17(2), pp.35-36.

Howe, E. 1980. Public Professions and the Private Mode of Professionalism, **Social Work**, 25(3), pp.179-191.

Hughes, E.C., Thorne, B., DeBaggis, A.M., Gurin A., and Williams, D. 1973. **Education for the Professions of Medicine, Law, Theology, and Social Welfare**. New York: McGraw-Hill.

Isenberg, S. and Cramond, D. 1986. Burying the Turf Issue, **The Next Step: The Glasrock Home Health Care Newsletter for Discharge Planning**, 3(1), July, pp.2-3.

Jannson, B.S. and Simmons, J. 1986. The Survival of Social Work Units in Host Organizations, **Social Work**, 32(5), pp.339-343.

Jette, A. 1983. Meeting the Needs of an Aging Population, **Health and Social Work**, 8(4), pp.325-330.

Joel, L. 1983. The State of the Art of Reimbursement for Nursing Services, **Nursing and Health Care**, 4, pp. 560-563.

Joint Commission for Accreditation of Hospitals (1979). **Manual for Accreditation of Hospitals.** Chicago. IL: American Hospital Association.

Johnson, J. 1975. **Doing Field Research.** New York: The Free Press.

Johnson, W.L. 1980. **Supply and Demand for Registered Nurses(Part I).** New York: National League for Nurses, Number 19-1837.

Kahn, A.J. 1959. **Issues in American Social Work.** New York: Columbia University Press.

Kahn, A.J. 1966. **Neighborhood Information Centers.** New York: Columbia University Press.

Kane, R.A. 1980. Discharge Planning: An Undischarged Responsibility, Editorial, **Health and Social Work,** 5, pp.2-3.

Kane, R.A. 1982. Lessons for Social Work from the Medical Model: A Viewpoint for Practice, **Social Work,** 27(4), pp.315-321.

Kane, R.A. 1983. Minding our PPOs and DRGs, **Health and Social Work,** 8, pp.82-84.

Kaplan, C. 1982. A Screening Grid for Hospital Counseling Services, **Health and Social Work,** 7(3), pp.220-223.

Kerson, T.S. 1979. Sixty Years Ago: Hospital Social Work in 1918, **Social Work in Health Care,** 4(3), pp.331-343.

Klegon, D. 1978. The Sociology of Professions: An Emerging Perspective, **Sociology of Work and Occupations,** 5(3), pp.259-283.

Kleyman, P. 1985. Community Services Burdened by DRGs, **Coordinator,** 4(9), pp.32-33.

Kligerman, M. J. and McKegney, F.P. 1971. Patterns of Psychiatric Consultation in Two General Hospitals, **International Journal of Psychiatry and Medicine**, 2, pp. 126-132.

Knowles, J. H. 1977. **Doing Better and Feeling Worse**. New York: W.W.Norton.

Kornblatt, E.S., Fisher, M.E. and MacMillan, D.J. 1985. Impact Of DRGs on Home Health Nursing, **QRB**, October, pp.290-294.

Krell, G.I. 1977. Overstay Among Hospital Patients: Problems and Approaches, **Health and Social Work**, 2, pp.163-178.

Kulys, R. 1983. Future Crisis of the Very Old: Implications for Discharge Planning, **Health and Social Work**, 8, pp.182-195.

Lacy, K.K. and McCulloch, E.S. 1982. Nursing Services. In **The Health Professions**. M.V. Boyles, M.K. Morgan, M.H. McCaulley, Eds. Philadelphia: W.B. Saunders Co.

Lee, A. Ed. 1984. 1984 and Beyond: What's Ahead for Nursing. **RN**. 47, pp. 26-29.

Levey, S. 1980. **Study of Hospital Discharges for Patients 65 and Over**. New York: Greater New York Hospital Association.

Lewis, H. 1982. The Emergence of Social Work as a Profession in Health Care: Significant Issues and Persistent Issues. In **Milestones in Social Work and Medicine**, H. Rehr, Ed. New York: Prodist.

Lindenberg, R.E. and Coulton, C. 1980. Planning for Post-Hospital Care: A follow-up Study, **Health and Social Work**, 5(1), pp.45-50.

Lipowsky, Z.J. 1967. Review of Consultation Psychiatry and Psychosomatic Medicine: II Clinical Aspects, **Psychosomatic Medicine**, 29, pp. 201-224.

Likert, R. 1961. **New Patterns of Management**. New York: McGraw-Hill.

Lowe, J. and Herranen, M. 1978. Conflicts in Teamwork: Understanding Roles and Relationships, **Social Work and Health Care**, 3(3), pp. 323-330.

Lurie, A., Pinsky, S., and Tuzman, L. 1981. Training Social Workers for Discharge Planning, **Health and Social Work**, 6(4), pp.12-18.

Lurie, A. and Rosenberg, G. 1984. **Social Work Administration in Health Care**. New York: Haworth Press.

Lysault, J.P. 1977. **An Abstract for Action**. New York: McGraw-Hill Co.

Magnusson, D. 1982. Situational Determinants of Stress. In **Handbook of Stress**, L. Goldberger and S. Breznitz (Eds.) New York: The Free Press.

Marshall, J.T. 1984. DRGs and the New Shape of Discharge Planning, **The Coordinator**, October, pp.16-22.

Mason, E.J. and Daugherty, J.K. 1984. Nursing tandards Should Determine Nursing's Price, **Nursing Management**, 15, pp. 34-38.

Mauksch, G. and David, M. 1972. Presciption for Survival, **American Journal of Nursing**, 72, pp. 2189-2193.

McCarthy, E. 1976. Comprehensive Home Care for Earlier Hospital Discharge, **Nursing Outlook**, 24 (10), pp. 625-630.

Mechanic, D. 1980. The Management of Psychosocial Problems in Primary Care: A Potential Role for Social Work, **Journal of Human Stress**, 6, pp. 16-21.

Mechanic, D. 1980. **Students Under Stress: A Study in Social Psychology of Adaptation.** Madison, WI: University of Wisconsin Press.

Medicare's Prospective Payment System: Strategies for Evaluation, Cost, Quality and Medical Technology. 1985 Washington, D.C.: Office of Technology Assessment.

Merton, R.K. 1957. **Social Theory and Social Structure.** New York: The Free Press.

Meyer, A. 1948. **The Commonsense Psychiatry.** New York: McGraw-Hill Book Co.

Meyer, C.H. 1981. Social Work Purpose: Status by Choice or Concern? **Social Work**, 26 (1), pp. 69-75.

Miller, R.D. and Rehr, H. 1983. **Social Work Issues in Health Care.** Englewood Cliffs, NJ: Prentice-Hall.

Miller-Allan, P. 1984. **Introduction to the Health Professions.** Monterey, CA: Wadsworth Health Science Division.

Mizrahi, T. 1988. Prospective Payments and Social Work: Obstacles and Opportunities. In **Innovations in Health Care Practice**, J.S. McNeil and S.E. Weinstein Eds. Silver Spring, Maryland: National Association of Social Workers.

Monk, A. 1981. Social Work with the Aged: Principles of Practice, **Social Work**, 26 (1), pp. 61-68.

Monk, A. and Stuen, C. 1988. **The Impact of Medicare's Prospective Payment System on Elderly Patients: A Study of Three New York City Hospitals.** New York: Columbia University. The Brookdale Institute on Aging and Adult Human Development.

Moore, W.E. 1970. **The Professions: Roles and Rules.** New York: Russell Sage Foundation.

Nason, F. and Delbanco, T. 1976. Soft Services: A Major Cost Effective Component of Primary Medical Care, **Social Work in Health Care,** 1(3).

National Association of Social Workers. 1977. **Standards for Hospital Social Services.** NASW Policy Statement, No. 6, Washington, DC: NASW.

National Center for Health Statistics. 1087. **Report to Congress: Impact of the Medicare Hospital Prospective Payment System,** Publication 03251. Baltimore: U.S. Dept. of Health and Human Services.

Office of Inspector General, Office of Analysis and Inspections. 1988. **National DRG Validation Study: Special Report on Premature Discharges.** OAI-05-88-00740. Washington, D.C.: Dept. of Health and Human Services, pp. i-ii.

Office of Technology Assessment, 1985. **Medicare's Prospective Payment System: Strategies for Evaluation, Cost, Quality and Medical Technology.** Washington, DC: Governmental Printing Office.

Olsen, K.M. and Olsen, M.E. 1967. Role Expectations and Perceptions for Social Workers in Medical Settings, **Social Work,** 12 (3), pp. 70-78.

Orem, D.E. 1980. **Nursing: Concepts of Practice.** 2nd Ed. New York: McGraw-Hill Co.

Ottinger, K.B. 1950. Why a Nurse Mental Health Consultant in Public Health, **Journal of Psychiatric Social Work**, 19, Spring.

Patchner, M.A. and Wattenberg, S.H. 1985. Impact of Diagnosis Related Groups on Hospital Social Service Departments, **Social Work**, 30 (3), pp. 259-261.

Payne, J.E. 1972. Ombudsman Roles for Social Work, **Social Work.** 17 (1), pp. 95-97.

Pearl, A. and Reissman, F. 1965. **New Careers for the Poor: The Non-Professional in Human Services.** New York: Free Press.

Pearlman, I.R. 1984. Discharge Planning: The Team is Behind You, **Nursing Management.** 15 (8), pp. 36-38.

Perretz, E. 1976. Social Work Education for the Field of Health, **Social Work in Health Care**, 1 (3), pp. 357-375.

Personal Communication with Bernard Danzig, President, Discharge Planning Association of New York City and Director of Social Services, Albert Einstein Hospital, Fall, 1985.

Personal Communication with Cynthia Roberti, Secretary, American Association of Continuity of Care, January, 1986.

Peterson, K.J. 1985. **Post-Hospital Needs and Adequacy of Resources for Patients Discharged to Multonah County.** Portland, OR: Regional Research Institute, Portland State University.

Pfouts, J.H. and McDaniel, B. 1977.
Medical Handmaidens or Professional
Colleagues, **Social Work in Health Care**,
2 (3), pp. 275-283.

Pilette, P.C. 1983. Overcoming the
Tyranny of Our Professional Role.
Nursing Management 14 (3). pp. 57-60.

Piper, L.R. 1983. Accounting for
Nursing Functions in DRGs, **Nursing
Management**, 14 (11), pp. 46-48.

Phillips, L. 1972. Hospital Discharge: by
Plan or by Chance? **Hospital Progress**,
53, pp. 23-26.

Polansky, N.A. 1975. **Social Work
Research**, Revised Edition. Chicago:
The University of Chicago Press.

Popple, P.R. 1986. The Social Work
Profession: A Reconceptualization,
Social Service Review, 59 (4), pp. 560-577.

Rademaker, A.J. 1982. **Technical Skills in
Registered Nursing and Related
Occupations**. Ann Arbor, MI:
University of Michigan Research Press.

Rasmusen, L.A. 1984. A Screening Tool
Promotes Early Discharge Planning,
Nursing Management, 15, pp. 39-42.

Ratliff, B.W., 1981. **Leaving the
Hospital: Discharge Planning for Total
Patient Care**. Springfield, IL:
Charles C. Thomas.

Reamer, F. G. 1985. Facing Up to the
Challenge of DRGs, **Health and Social
Work**, 10(2), pp. 85-94.

Regensberg, J. 1978. **Towards Education for
Health Professions**. New York: Harper
and Row, p.108.

Rehr, H.(Ed.) 1974. **Medicine and Social Work: An Expoloration in Interprofessionalism.** New York:Prodist.
Rehr, H. (Ed.), 1979. **Professional Accountability for Social Work Practice.** New York: Prodist.
Rehr, H. 1982. **Milestones in Social Work and Medicine.** New York: Prodist.
Rehr, H., Berkman, B., and Rosenberg, G. 1980. Screening for High Social Risk and Problems, **Social Work,** 25(5), pp.403-406.
Rehr, H. and Miller, R.S. 1983. More Issues for the Eighties. In **Social Work Issues in Health Care,** R. S. Miller and H. Rehr Eds. Englewood Cliffs, NJ: Prentice-Hall.
Reid, W.J. 1981. **Research in Social Work.** New York:Columbia University Press.
Robinson, S.S. 1967. Is There a Difference? **Nursing Outlook,** 15(11), pp. 34-36.
Rosenberg, G. and Rehr, H. (Eds.) 1982. **Advancing Social Work Practice in Health.** New York: Haworth Press.
Rossen, S. 1984. Adapting Discharge Planning to Prospective Pricing, **Hospitals,** March 1, pp.71-79.
Rothweiler, T.M. 1986. Does Education Affect Nursing Care? **Nursing Management,** 17 (4), pp.59-62.
Russell, L.B. 1989. **Medicare's New Hospital Payment System: Is it Working?** Washington, D.C.: The Brookings Institution.

Schaffer, F.A. 1984. A Nursing Perspective of the DRG World (Part I), **Nursing and Health Care**, 5(1), pp. 48-51.
Schaffer, F.A. 1984. Nursing Gearing Up for DRGs, Part II, Management Strategies, **Nursing and Health Care**, 5(2), pp. 93-99.
Schaffer, F.A. 1984. Nursing Power in the DRG World, **Nursing Management** 15, pp.28-30.
Schoenberg, B., Pettit, H.F., and Carr,A.C. (Eds.) 1968. **Teaching Psychosocial Aspects of Patient Care**. New York: Columbia University Press.
Schrager, J. 1971. Impediments to the Course and Effectiveness of Discharge Planning, **Social Work in Health Care**, 4, pp.65-77.
Schreiber, H. 1981. Discharge Planning: Key to the Future, **Health and Social Work**, 6, pp.48-53.
Schwartz, J. 1982. **Demographic Trends And Hospital Utilization: The Elderly Population**. Office of Public Policy Analysis, Policy Brief No. 41. Chicago, IL: American Hospital Association.
Selye, H. 1956. **The Stress of Life**. New York: McGraw Hill.
Seymour, L.R. 1954. **Selected Writings of Florence Nightengale**. New York: The MacMillan Company.
Sheppard-Towner Act, 1921, Chapter 135, 67th Congress.
Shulman, L. 1977. Social Work Education for Health Care Practice: Response to Professor Raymond, **Social Work in Health Care**, 2(4), pp.439-444.

Shulman, L. and Tuzman, L.1980. Discharge Planning-A Social Work Perspective, **Quality Review Bulletin**, 6(10), pp.3-8.
Siegel, S. 1956. **Nonparametric Statistics for the Behavioral Sciences.** New York: McGraw-Hill Company.
Singleton, E.K. and Nail, F.C.1984 Role Clarification: A Prerequisite to Autonomy. **The Journal of Nursing Administration**, 14(10), pp. 17-22.
Slepian, F.W. 1979. Medical Social Work in Primary Care, **Primary Care**, 6(3), pp.621-632.
Sloan, F.A., Morrisey, M.A., Valvona, J. 1988. Case Shifting and the Medicare Prospective Payment System. **American Journal of Public Health**, 78, pp. 553-556.
Social Work and the Challenge of DRGs, 1984. Editorial. **Health and Social Work**, 9(1), pp.2-3.
Soldo, B.J. and Agree, E.M. 1988. America's Elderly. **Population Bulletin**, 43(3). Population Reference Bureau, Washington, DC.
Specht, H., 1972. The Deprofessionalization of Social Work, **Social Work**, 17, pp. 3-15.
Stein, H.D. 1969. Reflections on Competence and Ideology in Social Work Education, **Journal of Education for Social Work**, 5(1), pp.81-90.
Stoeckle, J., Sittler, R. and Davidson, G. 1966. Social Work in a Medical Clinic: The Nature and Course of Referrals to the Social Worker, **American Journal of Public Health**, 56(9), pp.1570-1579.

Stoller, E.P. 1982. Sources of Support for the Elderly During Illness, **Health and Social Work**, 7(2), pp.111-122.

Suchman, E.A. 1965. Stages of Illness and Medical Care, **Journal of Health and Human Behavior**, 6, pp.114-128.

Swack, L.G. 1980. Education and Practice: Their Responsibility to Complement Each Other, **Health and Social Work**, 5(1), pp.64-70.

Toren, N. 1969. Semi-Professionalism and Social Work: A Theoretical Perspective. In **The Semiprofessions and Their Organization**, A. Etzioni, Ed. New York: The Free Press.

Toth, R.M. 1984. DRGs: Imperative Strategies for Nursing Service Administration, **Nursing and Health Care**, 5(4), pp. 197-203.

Turf Problem. 1984. Task Force Report. Washington, DC: American Association of Continuity of Care.

Ullman, A. and Kassebaum, G. 1961. Referrals and Service in a Medical Social Work Department, **Social Service Review**, 35, pp.258-267.

Ullman, A., Goss, M.E.W., Davis, M.S., and Mushinski, M. 1971. Activities, Satisfaction, and Problems of Social Workers in Hospital Settings: A Comparative Study, **Social Service Review**, 45, pp.17-29.

United Hospital Fund. 1986. **New Directions in Health Care: Consequences for the Elderly**. Paper Series 5, December.

Vladeck, B. 1985. Medicare Hospital Payment by Diagnosis Related Group, **Annals of Internal Medicine**, 100(4), pp.576-591.

Volland, P.J. 1988. **Discharge Planning: An Interdisciplinary Approach to Continuity of Care.** Owning Mills, MD: National Health Publishing.

Vollard, P. 1983. As cited in Irwin Reynolds, The National White House Briefing on Prospective Pricing of Medicare for Social Work Administrators: Preliminary Report to members of the Illinois Chapter of Society of Hospital Social Work Directors, Washington, DC, November 3-4.

Wallace, S.R., Goldberg, R.J. and Slaby, A.E. 1984. **Clinical Social Work in Health Care.** New York: Praeger.

Waters, V. 1965. Distinctions are Necessary, **American Journal of Nursing,** October, pp. 101-102.

Weil, M. Karls, J. and Associates. 1985. **Case Management in Human Services.** San Francisco: Jossey-Bass.

Wertheimer, D.S., Kleinman, L.S. 1990. A Model for Interdisciplinary Discharge Planning in a University Hospital. **The Gerontologist,** 30(6), pp. 837-840.

Wilensky, H.L. and Lebaux, C.N. 1965. **Industrial Society and Social Welfare.** New York: The Free Press.

Wilson, P.A. 1981. Expanding the Role of Social Workers in Coordination of Health Services, **Social Work,** 6(1), pp. 57-64.

Wilson, F.A. and Neuhauser, D. 1976. **Health Services in the United States.** Cambridge, MA: Ballinger.

Wolfbein, S. 1971. **Workers in American Society.** Glenview, IL: Scott, Foresman, and Company.
Yarmolinsky, A. 1978. What Future for the Professional in American Society? **Daedulus,** 107, pp.159-174.
Zimbalist, S. 1977. **Historic Themes and Landmarks in Social Welfare Research.** New York: Harper and Row.

Appendix

HOSPITAL SITE VISIT

"Social work's tradition of quantitative measurement and statistical computation of social problems has been steadfast from the late 1800's (Zimbalist, 1977). However there are limitations to quantitative measures, particularly the loss of more personal observations. Fortunately there is a resurgence of interest in qualitative methods of social research (Bogdan and Taylor, 1975). To this end, a site visit to one New York City hospital was conducted after the survey questionnaires had been returned and analyzed. The purpose of the site visit was to follow up some of the survey questions and findings with discharge planners, to obtain reactions about the impact of DRGs from other select hospital personnel, and obtain a more dynamic sense of changes in discharge planning in the acute care hospital setting during the past year to compensate for the limitations of survey research.

Site Selection

Three criteria were employed in selecting the hospital for a site visit. Auspice was important since the majority (67.5%) of acute care hospitals in New York City are not-for-profit. The second criteria was size. The most predominant hospital size in New York City is in the range of 200-399 beds. The final criteria was departmental responsibility for discharge planning. Since the variable of professional discipline is primary in the survey component of this study, it was deemed important to select a hospital where social workers and nurses are both engaged in discharge planning tasks within the same department.

A not-for-profit hospital was selected with a bed capacity between 200-399 and where the discharge planning unit was within the social work department. The social work department in this hospital is known as the 'Social Work/Discharge Planning Department' and employs both nurses and social workers. It is referred to as Hospital A to protect the anonymity of respondents.

The organization table for Hospital A's Social Work/Discharge Planning Department is provided in Table A-1. The Director of Social Work who leads this department is a certified social worker with the additional title of Discharge Planning Coordinator. The director reports to the hospital's Associate Director for Financial Services. Table A-2 identifies the administrative table of organization for Hospital A. It is noteworthy that the Social Work/Discharge Planning Department along with the departments of Patient Review (DRG Coordination), Utilization Review, and Admitting are supervised by the Associate Director of Financial Services. This supervisor also has responsibility for the departments of Engineering, Maintenance, and Purchasing. This places an obvious financial emphasis on the social work/discharge planning services.

Site Visit Protocol

The purpose of the site visit was to provide a more qualitative sense of the new climate resulting from prospective reimbursement and its particular effect on discharge planning. It was not conceived as

Hospital Site Visit

Table A-1
SOCIAL WORK/DISCHARGE PLANNING DEPARTMENT

Table of Organization

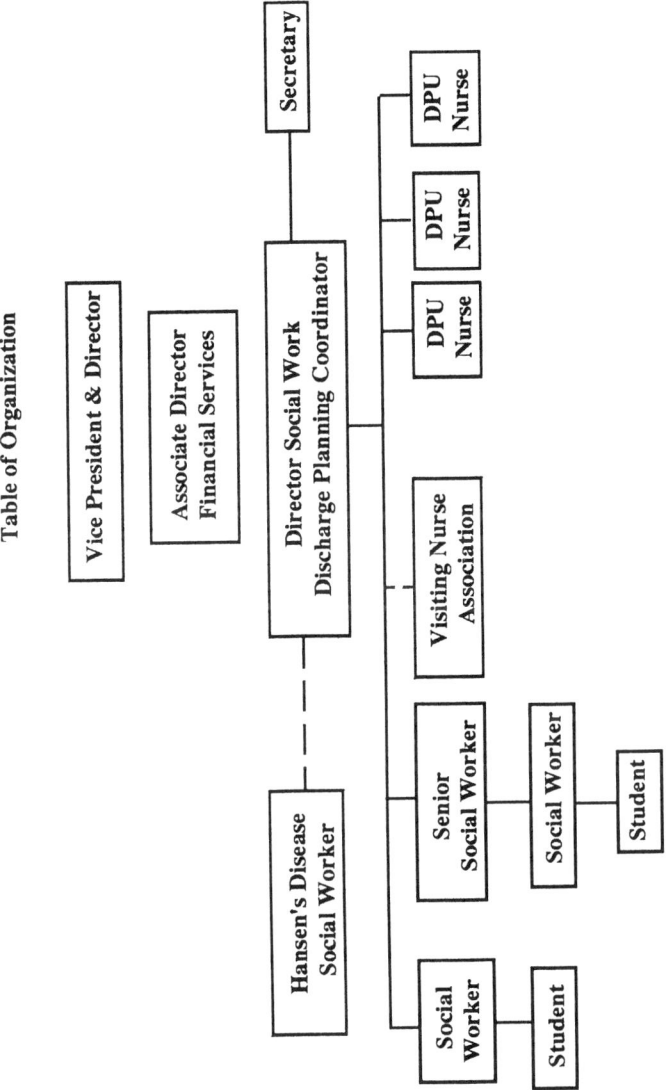

TABLE A-2
HOSPITAL A
August, 1986
TABLE OF ORGANIZATION

Vice President & Director	**Associate Director, Financial Services**

Cancer Support Coordinator
Community Relations/
  Volunteers
Medical Staff
Pastoral Care
Q.A. Physician Advisor
Training Director
  (P.A. School)
	Admitting/PAT
	Engineering/Maintenance
	Finance (all areas)
	Gift Shop
	Patient Review (DRG)
	Purchasing
	Social Work/Discharge Planning
	Utilization Review

Deputy Director	**, Assistant Director**
Alcohol Detoxification Anesthesiology Gynecology Infection Control Medicine/all sub-specialities Medical Library Pathology/Laboratory Pharmacy Psychiatry/Inpt. & Outpt. Quality Assurance Radiology/Nuclear Medicine Rehabilitation Respiratory Care Services Risk Management Surgery/all sub-specialities SUSSI	CHAMPUS/Military Liaison ER/Outpatient Clinics Mecial Records New Lane Project Speech/Hearing
	Associate Director, Nursing
	Ambulatory Surgery Food & Nutrition Nursing Administration Nursing Education OPD/ER Nursing Operating Room Patient Care Areas Patient Transport Services Renal Dialysis
, Asst. Dir.	**Director, Human Resources**
Building Services Central Sterile Supply Communications/Info desk Materials Management Storeroom/Reproduction	Employee Health Mail Room Patient Relations Personnel Security Tonsorial Services Transportation

a rigorous case study but rather an opportunity to confirm quantitative data findings among discharge planning personnel. To probe non-discharge planning personnel in Administration, and the departments of Utilization Review, Quality Assurance, Patient Review (DRG Coordination), and the Geriatric Primary Care Clinic. Seven questions were formulated based on the original research objectives that were generically appropriate to the various departments identified. Clearance for meeting with staff in each department/division was obtained and a memorandum (approved by administration) was circulated by the Director of Social Work/Discharge Planning to all target personnel one week in advance of the site visit.

The primary method of input was personal interview conducted either in small groups or individually. A secondary method of input was written responses to the seven questions. An overview of data sources and method of input follows.

Hospital Data Source/(Method of Input)
Executive Director/(1)
Assoc. Director of Finance/(1)
Director of Planning/(2)
Utilization Review Coordinator/(3)
Quality Assurance Coordinator/(3)
Patient Review Director/(3)
Director of Social Work/(2)
Discharge Planning Coor./(1)
Social Workers/(3)
Nurses in Discharge Planning Unit/(3)
VNA Nurse Assigned to Hospital/(3)
Nurse Practitioners in Geriatric Primary Care Clinic/(2)

180 Appendix

Key:
(1)Written Reply; (2)Individual Interview; (3)Group Interview
Each of the seven questions are stated below and responses summarized. When respondents from the various departments/divisions differed, the areas of variance are reported. When interviewees respond similarly, data are summarized across disciplines.

Question 1: *What are your opinions about the Prospective Payment System (DRGs) for Medicare eligible patients?*

All respondents had both positive and negative opinions about DRGs. The positive comments, among all but the two nurse practitioners in the geriatric primary care clinic, were expressed in terms of health care cost. All respondents mentioned areas of waste or unnecessary expense prior to the implementation of the Prospective Payment System (January, 1986). The Executive Director and Associate Director for Financial Services cited increased efficiency in the areas of test procedures ordered for patients as well as their timely completion.

The Utilization Review and Quality Assurance personnel felt there had been a lot of waste during the period of retrospective reimbursement and that money could be saved appropriately in the new system. A second positive outcome attributed to PPS was an increased focus on continuing education for all hospital personnel. Physicians are now being reprimanded for inefficient treatment, being educated in the DRG system, and modifying their practice accordingly.

Nurses engaged in discharge planning experienced physicians as most angry about the changes concomitant with DRG implementation. The nurses felt physicians had taken advantage of the retrospective payment system and the new system, while taking some adjustment, was basically a good idea. Social workers recognized the iatrogenic effects of hospitalization on older persons and recognized that sometimes a 'quicker' discharge was positive. Social workers, in surprising contrast with survey findings, were the only group to mention that the discharge planning functions, since DRGs, had enhanced their status among hospital personnel.

Many negative opinions about DRGs were shared. The Executive Director felt that one negative outcome of PPS was the fiscal instability created for some hospitals. This resulted in several closings in the past year. Another negative expressed by social workers and discharge planning nurses was related to the lack of a community-based continuum of care available to the older adults who were being discharged 'quicker and sicker.' The discharge planning nurses also cited the cutbacks in Medicare coverage for home care benefits enacted at the same time DRGs were implemented which created many hardships for patients. Social workers observed that 'DRG-induced panic' among physicians had bred inconsistent treatment for patients. A negative iatrogenic effect of hospitalization on the elderly was expressed by social workers. Taking a 90 year old woman admitted for a heart condition who spends five days in bed, most likely needs some physical therapy to overcome the lack of mobility but the new

DRG methodology does not take into account this kind of need often seen among the elderly. A double bind is now created. The hospital cannot justify keeping the patient just for physical therapy while at the same time Medicare will not cover physical therapy in the community for her diagnosed heart condition. The patient has to pay for physical therapy out of pocket and may or may not have the means to do so.

The lack of individual differences within each DRG was of concern to the geriatric nurse practitioners who follow up discharged elderly patients in the community. Some elderly patients do need more time in the hospital in order for their return home to work out well. Quality assurance and utilization review interviewees also cited this loss of the 'human factor.'

One overwhelmingly positive statement was expressed by most staff in the midst of their discussion of the negative impacts of DRGs. That was their hospital's philosophy of care, "put the patient first." If a patient really needed to stay in the hospital, administration was sensitive and supportive.

Question 2: *What changes, if any, has Hospital A made in its operation since DRGs went into effect?*

Several respondents cited computerization as a by-product of the new Prospective Payment System. This has contributed to increased efficiency. Administration, with the computerized billing information, now identifies 'good' and 'bad' physicians. The criterion for a 'bad' physician is simple, their patients lose money for the hospital. Top administrators are given a routine summary 'hit list of the bad physicians.' While the two administrators acknowledge this is simplistic, it has served to at least moderate the behavior of ordering unnecessary tests and performing unnecessary and costly procedures.

Utilization review/quality assurance personnel cited an increased use of pre-admission testing and day surgery as a result of DRGs and felt it positive. This group of personnel also stated their belief that there was no increase in the rate of readmission among the elderly at their hospital in the past year. This is a definite contradiction with the perception of discharge planners in the survey research findings.

Social workers indicated a change in the alternate level of care status (ALOC). In their hospital, the ALOC days have greatly decreased. They attribute this to the impact Resource Utilization Groupings are having on nursing home admissions. The patient requiring more skilled nursing who was kept in the hospital awaiting nursing home placement, is now being accepted more readily. In addition, social work developed a system of direct delivery of applications to nursing homes rather than waiting for postal delivery.

The hiring of a Director of Patient Review is a very visible sign of change attributed to DRGs. The title is a euphemism for DRG Coordinator. This person's job is to educate staff about DRGs and monitor the lengths of stay and utilization of resources by patients. DRG management is a new concept in hospitals but a rapidly expanding one as evidenced by the establishment of a new professional organization, the DRG Management Association of New York. This association is open to 'professionals involved in or concerned with DRGs.'

Another very visible personnel change is the provision of a staff person by each borough's Visiting Nurse Association. This person, a nurse, is located in the discharge planning unit among the nurses, and accepts referrals for visiting nurse and/or rehabilitative care. The nurse insures that needed patient services from the Visiting Nurse Service begin on the day of discharge from the hospital.

The area of communication enhancement was mentioned by administration, social workers, nurses and nurse practitioners as a change. The respondents universally reported increased communication among disciplines since the new Prospective Payment System became effective. While agreeing, the geriatric nurse practitioners raised one concern, in spite of increased communication, ageism was still a deterrent to rehabilitative care for older persons among health care professionals.

The Director of Planning and Development reported that the recognition of service delivery and its costs were now more closely associated since DRGs went into effect. He thought this was a favorable change in that it has brought a new sense of financial consciousness to all levels of hospital staff, particularly physicians.

Question 3: *Do you think all patients will eventually be covered by a prospective reimbursement method?*

All respondents, individually and in groups, agreed that all patients will eventually be covered by a prospective reimbursement system. The three top administrators also gave a date. They cited information from the New York State Department of Health indicating that all providers of health care in acute care hospitals will be reimbursed prospectively by 1988. In addition the Executive Director and Associate Director for Finance pointed out that the bureaucracy of two methods of reimbursement in operation now, the one for Medicare patients and one for non-Medicare patients, is neither logical nor efficient.

Question 4: *Do you think discharge planning with the elderly has changed since DRGs went into effect?*

Administrators commented that discharge planning was already changing prior to DRGs, as a consequence of increased regulations by Professional Review Organizations (PROs) and required utilization review procedures, but has continued to change since PPS implementation. It was acknowledged by administration that the time constraints are more stringent now and that this has created more stress for discharge planning personnel. The Director of Planning and Development labeled the change in discharge planning with the elderly as an 'increased burden' for discharge planners, and pointed out that the greatest change needed was in the area of physician education. The goal of discharge planning with the elderly has remained unchanged, 'to develop and follow through on an organized plan of post-hospital care.'

Discharge planning nurses indicated that staff size in discharge planning has increased since DRGs and that staff awareness of the discharge planning functions has increased as well. Social workers in discharge planning felt they had to be more creative and work faster since DRGs to accomplish timely discharge plans. As mentioned previously, hand delivery of nursing home applications and the willingness of nursing homes to admit 'more skilled-need patients' are two specific changes attributable to the Prospective Payment System.

A FAX machine (computerized data facsimile transfer) is enabling instantaneous transfer of information to nursing homes and regulatory agencies. It's use is very helpful especially given the 'sicker' condition in which patients are transferred to nursing homes and the need for expedited Medicaid approval.

Question 5: *Do you think there are adequate community based and institutional resources available to meet elderly patient's needs?*

Utilization review/quality assurance personnel believed that while resources in the community are not as limited as they once were, considerable expansion is still needed. Administration, while agreeing with the lack of resources, did recognize the positive impact which Resources Utilization Groupings (RUGs) has had on nursing home availability. Patients in need of skilled nursing home care are no longer languishing in the hospital for weeks awaiting admission to a nursing home. Administration did point out that there were new categories of patients, some elderly and some not, for whom there are few community resources. The homeless were cited as an illustration of this particular problem area. While the homeless are not necessarily related to DRG reimbursement, their shelter is a needed community resource not adequately available. Social workers identified a lack of affordable homemaker and home health aide services. If a patient has adequate private means, community based resources can be purchased, but Medicare cutbacks in home care service coverage has created a real deficit in home support services for the elderly who are less well off. Medicaid is an important community resource and there have been positive improvements in its management to reduce the time of application and approval, however, Medicaid which will cover in home services only affects 20% of the elderly. This leaves a large group of elderly, primarily middle and lower middle class people quite vulnerable when returning to the community.

Nurses in the discharge planning unit were very negative about the adequacy of community resources availability. Inaccessible and inadequate were the best descriptors of their reactions.

Question 6: *What role do you think hospitals should have in the development of services for the elderly?*

With one exception, all respondents were overwhelmingly in favor of the hospital initiating and developing services for the elderly. Social workers viewed the hospital as the hub of care and other staff supported the need for the hospital being involved in an expansion of the continuity of care resources. Administration, while agreeing that the hospital has a role in the development of services, saw it primarily for its marketing potential. Former patients or potential patients served well by a hospital affiliated community resource may be more likely to use that hospital when needed. The Director of Planning and Development recognized the vested interest of the hospital in developing services in the community, including non health-related types of services e.g., housing.

The one group of respondents who were less positive about the hospital's role in developing services for the elderly was discharge planning nurses. They express concern that the hospital cannot do it all and thought there should be a broader base of community involvement in developing such services.

Question 7: *Do you find elderly patients appealing discharge decisions more frequently since DRGs?*

In Hospital A there have been no formal appeals of discharge decisions by elderly patients or their families on their behalf since DRGs went into effect. There have been situations which came close to an official action but, usually through the intervention of social workers with the patient and family, the administration and the patient's physician, appeals have been avoided.

Social workers spoke of what they called a generation of elderly who are 'physician-compliant.' If the 'doctor says it, that must be best' is the prevailing attitude. There is little general awareness of DRGs and the fiscal constraints which encourage the hospital to discharge patients more quickly than in the past and little resistance to physician decisions. However, the discharge planning nurses felt the major problem in situations nearing an appeals point was lack of communication on the part of physicians, sometimes with the patient and sometimes with the hospital team members.

The hospital's philosophy of caring for the patient prevails. Patients is Hospital A are not put out of the hospital if it is not in their best interest, DRGs or not.

Question specific to nurses and social workers in discharge planning.

The variable of professional discipline was very important in the data analysis of the survey research, therefore an additional area of inquiry was probed when the researcher met with discharge planning nurses and social workers. The overall response to questioning on the complementarity of social workers and nurses working in discharge planning was affirmative. The Director of Social Work reported that while nurses were initially suspect of a social worker being 'in charge,' a real sense of collegiability has developed. The director attributed the success of teamwork to clearly defined job descriptions, which delineate the roles for each discipline.

A strategy that has worked well for the director in working out turf problems has been to utilize staff meetings for case discussions. The strategy is simple: whomever has the best relationship with the patient, regardless of discipline, is given the authority to take leadership responsibility with the patient calling on the skills of colleagues as needed.

Nurse respondents were generally very positive about the ability of nurses and social workers to work together. The nurses felt appreciated for their unique contribution in understanding a patient's medical and nursing needs as well as the degree of patient education required for patients to resume as much independence as possible.

Nurses working in the discharge planning division of the department of social work continue to identify as 'nurses.' They do have a strong identification with their profession although they feel their role is not well understood by the more traditional nurses who provide direct patient care. Nurses did cite one area of role confusion or role blurring with social workers, high risk screening. Both nurses and social workers believe themselves to be uniquely trained to conduct high risk screening and occasionally this results in duplication of effort.

One frustration among social workers, also revealed in the survey results is the diminishment of the counseling role; their work is mostly crisis intervention in nature. Given the limited hospital stay of patients and the increased workload on social workers, if a patient does require psychosocial counseling, a referral must be made for others to follow up after discharge.

The impression of the researcher is that nurses and social workers are partners in this hospital, recognizing and respecting the unique contributions of each others discipline, and they are not so threatened by turf issues that the patient is lost sight of in the process. Clearly the climate created by prospective payment is one with little time for turf battles to interfere with discharge planning functions and fortunately few occur in this hospital.

In summary, responses from this site-visit Hospital confirmed the survey findings that discharge planners are under more severe time constraints to carry out their functions. The opinion that eventually all patients will be covered by a prospective form of reimbursement was confirmed.

While not asked directly about personnel's responsibility to advise and inform consumers of the appeals mechanism, it was clear from interaction with staff that they viewed their jobs from the host-agency perspective. It is their job to prevent appeals or resolve problems which could result in appeals, not to advise patients of their rights. Discharge planning nurses were the only group to confirm the survey findings that discharge planning staff size had increased as a consequence of DRGs. The specificity of changes associated with DRGs which included the computerization and its uses; and messenger delivery of applications to nursing homes were uncovered by the site visit. This enhanced the researcher's understanding of the various changes attributable to DRGs.

High risk screening is conducted by social work department staff according to 90% of survey respondents however it was the one area of role duplication mentioned by the discharge planning nurses. Both social workers and discharge planning nurses do high risk screening as mandated by New York State Health Department regulations and nurses judged themselves to be significantly more involved than the study revealed.

The site visit findings differed from the survey results in a few areas. One was the recognition of more positive response associated with the Prospective Payment System. Interviewees questioned the charge of inefficiency in the retrospective from of reimbursement. Discharge planners responding to the survey did not feel that a prospective form of reimbursement would make the hospital more efficient.

Social workers interviewed at Hospital A did feel their role was enhanced by DRGs whereas this was less true among the survey respondents in the same profession. Social workers also expressed concern about iatrogenic effects of the hospital environment on the elderly however in the survey responses, both nurses and social workers agreed that sometimes it is better to be 'discharged quicker and sicker.'

In response to questioning on the adequacy of community based and institutional services, none of staff queried reported case management as an unmet service need. This need had emerged among survey respondents as dramatically increased since the implementation of DRGs.

Hospital interviews documented both positive and negative changes of DRGs while basically reflecting a responsible attitude of caring for the whole person and not succumbing to rigid fiscal constraints at a patient's expense. The site visit raised several areas for further research. Central to these was the relationship between the departmental leadership of discharge planning units and discharge planners' sense of collegiality, job satisfaction and communication.